A Handbook of Drug Training

Clear, concise and practical, *A Handbook of Drug Training* is intended for people who run training events about drugs and working with drug users. It will be invaluable for informing others who know little or nothing about drugs, and for helping to develop the skills of those working with drug users.

Written from a holistic and humanistic perspective, the handbook provides a set of guidelines for doing drug training, and emphasises the importance of practice-based training courses. Extensive and practical, the book includes chapters on attitudes, drugs and their effects, harm reduction, critical incidents, stress management, and training the trainers, explaining why each topic is significant to drug training. Each chapter includes sample exercises and course designs that can be used in planning learning events.

Designed primarily for trainers and practitioners in the drug, AIDS and alcohol fields, *A Handbook of Drug Training* will also be relevant and useful to non-specialists and to students of the helping and caring professions.

Dave Macdonald and **Vicky Patterson** have worked in continuing adult education, and with drug users in both the statutory and voluntary sectors. For the past six years, as training organisers, they have developed the Drugs Training Project at the University of Stirling.

A Handbook of Drug Training

Learning About Drugs and Working
with Drug Users

Dave Macdonald
and
Vicky Patterson

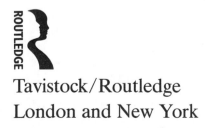

Tavistock/Routledge
London and New York

First published in 1991
by Routledge
11 New Fetter Lane, London EC4P 4EE

Simultaneously published in the USA and Canada
by Routledge
a division of Routledge, Chapman and Hall Inc.
29 West 35th Street, New York, NY 10001

© 1991 Dave Macdonald and Vicky Patterson
Typeset in Times Roman by Leaper & Gard Ltd, Bristol
Printed and bound in Great Britain by
Biddles Ltd, Guildford and King's Lynn

British Library Cataloguing in Publication Data
Macdonald, Dave *1946–*
  A handbook of drug training: learning about drugs and
  working with drug users.
  1. Great Britain. Drug abuse. Prevention and treatment
  I. Title II. Patterson, Vicky *1949–*
  362.29370941

Library of Congress Cataloging in Publication Data
Macdonald, Dave, 1946–
  A handbook of drug training: learning about drugs and working
  with drug users/Dave Macdonald and Vicky Patterson.
  p.   cm.
  Includes bibliographical references.
  Includes index.
  1. Narcotic addicts – Rehabilitation – Study and teaching.   2. Drug
  abuse – Health aspects. 3. Health education. I. Patterson, Vicky.
  1949–   . II. Title.
  [DNLM: 1. Health Education. 2. Social Work – education.
  3. Substance Abuse. 4. Substance Abuse – rehabilitation.
  5. Voluntary Workers – education. WM 270 M135h]
  RC564.M23 1991
  362.29–dc20
  DNLM/DLC
  for Library of Congress   90–9141
                                                             CIP

ISBN 0–415–06171–7
ISBN 0–415–04123–6 (Pbk)

For Graham, Liz and Roseanna

Contents

Figures and tables

FIGURES

TABLES

Acknowledgements

We would like to acknowledge the following people for their contributions to this handbook – Mike Ashton, Annas Dixon, Dr James Hawkins, Dr Peter Honey and Allan Mumford, Tony Manning and Dr Antony Thorley for allowing us to include their material; Andy Fox for co-writing Chapter 7 on 'harm reduction'; Robin Hall for co-designing the original Groupwork Course; Dr James Hawkins for his presentations and ideas on the Stress Management Workshop; David Pattison for co-designing the Critical Incidents Course. These three training courses were the foundation for the corresponding chapters in this handbook.

Ali Chalmers, Breda Flaherty, Colin Gilmour and Graham Walkinshaw for reading and commenting on the manuscript in its various stages of development; Anna Buchanan for typing the manuscript on our antiquated word processor; Duncan McKendrick and Graham Walkinshaw for the photographs on p. 18; Rosemary Nixon and Gill Davies, our editors from Routledge for their non-interventionist editing style.

There are of course many other people who have given us ideas, inspiration, suggestions, encouragement and support. A special thanks to Annas Dixon, Bob Dylan, Liz Kemp, Jan Le Flohic, Nelson Mandela and the many participants who shared the training courses and workshops with us. Thank you.

Introduction – how to use this handbook

This handbook is intended primarily for all those people putting on training events about drugs and working with drug users. These training events cover two major areas:

1 Enhancement of knowledge for those people who have little or no knowledge about drugs and drug users.
2 Skills development through experiential and participatory learning for those people working with drug users.

We envisage the handbook being particularly relevant to the following groups of people – educators on qualifying courses for the caring professions, e.g. Diploma in Social Work, Nursing Studies; in-service training courses for professional groups dealing with drug users including social workers, prison officers, community education workers, probation officers, youth and community workers; drug workers putting on learning events for volunteer counsellors, parents and families, interdisciplinary and community groups; addiction counsellors and those moving from the alcohol field into the broader field of drug work; teachers and lecturers in schools and post-school education; HIV and AIDS educators and trainers; the consumers of training, i.e. anybody who attends a training event on a drug-related topic.

How you use this handbook will depend on what you are looking for and who you are, for example, you may be a trainer/educator about to enter the drug field or a drug worker about to start training other workers, volunteers, or community groups. Whatever specific aspect of drug training you are interested in we would recommend that you first read Chapter 1 on training methods and approaches, which raises a number of key issues and questions and provides a set of guidelines for doing drug training.

The handbook is not meant to be prescriptive; rather its purpose is to help stimulate ideas for training. It provides several course structures and exercises that you can use for planning future learning events. These are 'ideal' courses and exercises that you should adapt according to your circumstances and available resources.

Note that each chapter is not structured in a similar way, although each does define what the topic is, why it is important for drug work and how to go about doing training in this area. This is intentional and reflects the fact that there is no one training-course model that each topic can be neatly fitted into. People who are only interested in reading about one particular topic will benefit from reading about other topics as they will discover different ideas in each chapter which will enhance the training they intend to do. For example, Chapter 4 includes more ideas and exercises on introductions, support and evaluation than any other chapter.

The handbook is set out in a way which generally reflects the learning experience as a continuous process which starts with attitudes, moves to knowledge and information enhancement and then to skills development. It focuses on building on the knowledge, information and skills that people already have.

Chapter 2 provides several exercises to enable course participants to examine their attitudes to drugs and drug users. It also says *why* this is an important first step in drug training.

Chapter 3 goes on to look at several different methods of teaching people about drugs and their effects and how to make an information-giving session like this as interesting as possible.

Chapters 4 and 5 provide training-course models that are oriented more towards the personal development and therefore wellbeing of the worker. Although the two areas – stress management and support systems, and groupwork – are relevant to a wide range of workers in the caring professions, it is shown why these two areas have particular significance for those working with drug users.

Chapters 6 and 7 provide training-course models that are designed to enable drug workers to gain, or enhance, skills in dealing with critical incidents and health-related problems and developing harm-reduction strategies.

Chapter 8, 'Training the trainers', gives a step-by-step account of how to train other people to develop a basic drug-awareness course.

Other areas and skills important for working with drug users have not been included in any depth because they have been adequately covered elsewhere, e.g. assessment, understanding the drug user, relapse (Dixon, 1987; Griffiths and Pearson, 1988; Shephard, 1990). Anyone working with drug users should already have a knowledge of basic counselling skills. For this reason we have chosen to include a chapter on the often neglected topic of groupwork rather than a basic counselling course. There are several good training manuals currently available on counselling (Egan, 1981; Egan, 1982; Inskipp, 1983; Woolfe, 1989).

This book only includes *basic* skills for learning about drugs and working with drug users. The Drugs Training Project, for example, offers a wide range of more specialised training such as team development work with individual drug projects; courses for or including managers and management committees; courses for administrative and secretarial staff on 'Working on the Front Line'; and courses for specific types of drug workers, e.g. detached workers, residential workers. Subject-specific courses are also part of a skills development programme for drug workers, e.g. 'Working with Families'; 'Working with Women'; 'Working with the Chronically Sick'; 'Loss and Bereavement'.

When we refer to a learning event or training course in the text this means any situation that is organised and structured to facilitate learning. It could mean anything from a 1-day workshop or seminar to a 3- or 4-day course which could be residential or non-residential.

When we refer to a 'trainer' in the text this applies to someone who may be a teacher, facilitator or other type of group leader.

When we refer to 'drugs' in the text this means all types of psychoactive substances, including those that are legal, those that are illegal and those that can be used both legally and illegally. The drug training in this handbook, however, has developed from work done in what is known as the drug field rather than the alcohol field, emphasising those drugs other than legal substances like alcohol and nicotine. The Drugs Training Project at Stirling University is funded by the Scottish Home and Health Department and was established in 1984 to offer education, training and support to drug workers and social work departments throughout Scotland. The major part of the work has been to design and run courses for drug workers and volunteers in both the voluntary and statutory sectors, particularly those who are working with intra-venous drug users.

It should be noted that there is not a separate chapter on HIV and AIDS. Rather these and related topics have been integrated into each chapter where appropriate. Dealing with issues surrounding HIV and AIDS is now everyday work for many drug workers, particularly those working with intravenous drug users. The shock waves caused by HIV and AIDS have caused a ripple effect that has resonated from drug user to worker to trainer. Anyone doing training for drug workers, for example, needs to acknowledge and deal with how these shock waves affect them before starting any training event (Cranfield and Dixon, 1990).

REFERENCES

Cranfield, S. and Dixon, A. (1990) *Drug Training, HIV and AIDS in the 1990s – A Guide for Training Professionals,* London: HEA.

Dixon, A. (1987) *Dealing with Drugs,* London: BBC Publications.

Egan, G. (1981) *The Skilled Helper: A Model for Systematic Helping and Interpersonal Relating,* Monterey, CA: Brooks/Cole.

Egan, G. (1982) *Exercises in Helping Skills,* Monterey, CA: Brooks/Cole.

Griffiths, R. and Pearson, B. (1988) *Working With Drug Users,* London: Wildwood House.

Inskipp, F. (1983) *A Manual for Trainers – A Resource Book for Setting Up and Running Basic Counselling Courses,* Alexia Publications.

Shephard, A. (1990) *Substance Dependency: A Professional Guide,* Birmingham: Venture Press.

Woolfe, R. (1989) *Counselling Skills: A Training Manual,* Edinburgh: SHEG.

Chapter 1

Training methods and approaches

This chapter is intended to set a basic framework for the rest of the book. It will raise a number of questions and issues and provide a set of guidelines for doing drug training. These are not meant to be prescriptive but to raise awareness and generate ideas; it is the task of each individual trainer to work out the approach that suits them best.

There are many different philosophies, models and theories of training and what we are offering here is the approach that has worked best for us in our work as drug trainers and for the drug workers who have been participants on our training events.

While the theoretical background to training is important, we should also acknowledge that training, like any other type of work with people, has an *intuitive* side which is often forgotten. For example, just as many social workers use intuitive skills in their work (Brandon, 1976; England, 1986) so a drug trainer should listen to his or her own feelings and personal insights about people and learning situations as well as to theories and models. Intuition, or what Polanyi calls 'tacit knowledge', is by definition an intangible quality that is difficult to measure or evaluate yet it is seen increasingly as an important influence on human behaviour (Assagioli, 1971; Blakeslee, 1980; Polanyi, 1983).

This book is written from a perspective we call 'well-worker training', which means that a priority of training should be the personal development, and therefore wellbeing, of the worker. If a worker feels confident, assured and supported, as well as practically skilled and informed, then they will be much more able to cope in working with drug users. For example, if a worker is skilled in counselling techniques but feels unsupported or insecure about working in a staff team or with a management committee and is having difficulties in coping with the pressures of work, then this will detrimentally affect the service provided to the client.

There are two specific sets of ideas which inform our approach to drug training that you should consider before planning a training event or reading further within this handbook about substantive training areas.

THE LEARNING SITUATION – TRAINING OR EDUCATION?

It is necessary to be aware of what we are doing to, doing for, or doing with people in the learning situation. Quite often what is called 'training' lies somewhere on a continuum between training and education, and not at either extreme. In the drug field, as elsewhere, the learning situation should be an appropriate mix between training and its opposite and contradictory concept – education (see Figure 1.1). When we use the word 'training' in this book we are talking about this mix, rather than the more rigid definition of training used in Figure 1.1.

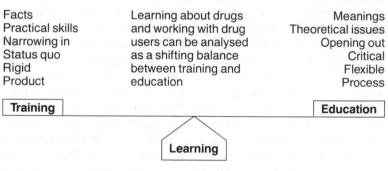

Facts	Learning about drugs	Meanings
Practical skills	and working with drug	Theoretical issues
Narrowing in	users can be analysed	Opening out
Status quo	as a shifting balance	Critical
Rigid	between training and	Flexible
Product	education	Process

| Training | | Education |

Learning

Source: Macdonald, 1989:9.

Figure 1.1   The balance between training and education

Training, as illustrated in Figure 1.1 means looking at facts and providing practical skills for dealing with them. It implies obedience and that there is a 'right' and a 'wrong' way of doing things. It is often more rigid than education, being based on the status quo and promising an end product i.e. the trained or skilled worker. 'Training involves a *narrowing down* of the consciousness to master certain techniques or skills' (Abbs, 1987).

Education, on the other hand, looks at the meanings behind the facts and the issues that arise from them, as well as the facts themselves. Ideally, it should be a critical flexible process valid in itself whether or not there is an end product such as skills or qualifications. 'Education is an *opening out* of the mind which transcends detail/skill and whose movement cannot be predicted' (Abbs 1987).

From these definitions it is clear that what many people bring to a learning event on drugs is their experience of training, not education. This may be their experience of a school system which fits the criteria for training rather than education, and which is typically based on a didactic top-down approach that rarely allows its participants to negotiate their own learning needs or empowers them to be responsible for their own learning. Even professional training courses, e.g. in social work, teaching or medicine, which may to an extent empower students, will rarely allow them to negotiate their own learning needs. As a result many people attending a learning event on drugs may expect to be provided with the facts about drugs and drug users and the practical skills to deal with them – end of story!

However, note that education by itself is as limited as training by itself in helping people to cope through their learning about drug problems. It can be so woolly that it never tackles the issues it discusses in a practical sense. What is needed is an appropriate mix of training and education. If education is emphasised rather than the training product, for example, people may initially feel deskilled and *less* able to cope, because they feel their existing knowledge base and skills are inadequate, and no new skills have been learnt. They may feel personally challenged or criticised. However, their competence will eventually be enhanced as they discover how to adapt their existing skills to the issues that emerge during the learning experience – learning *how* to solve their problems rather than just what the solutions are. Indeed, many educational models assume that learning is an exploratory process filled with tension and conflict and therefore needs to be conducted within a context of safety and support. This section was first published in *Druglink* (Macdonald 1989).

The model in Figure 1.1 can be used as a checklist so that you are aware of the *balance* in any learning situation between training and education. The balance itself will depend on the aims and objectives of the training event that have already been negotiated

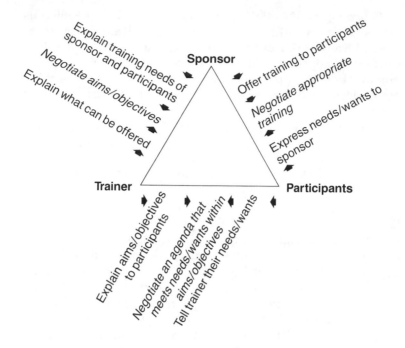

Source: Dixon and Gordon, 1987:2.

Figure 1.2   Organising a training event: the negotiation process

with all those involved – sponsor, trainers and participants. These aims and objectives will vary according to people's needs and agendas, their background and their level of knowledge and experience in working with drug users. You can think about this negotiation process in terms of a triangle (see Figure 1.2). This negotiation process can be complex and time-consuming, although time spent at this stage is invaluable in preparing the groundwork for a successful training event. Here are some questions to consider when entering into this process:

1 Is the training proactive or reactive? Are you initiating the training or are you responding to a request from an individual or an organisation, a sponsor or a participant?
2 Are you negotiating mainly with workers/participants or managers/sponsors? Whose needs are being met, those of indi-

viduals or those of the organisation? How will you find out what participants' needs are?

3 Will participants be coming to the training event on a voluntary or involuntary basis? What effect could this have?

4 Are there any hidden agendas from the participants or sponsors that will adversely affect the negotiating process *or* the training event?

The following section provides some of the information you will need to take into account when entering into this negotiation process and planning a learning event.

A HOLISTIC AND HUMANISTIC APPROACH TO LEARNING

The notion of 'holistic' is currently enjoying a revival, particularly in the fields of health and medicine (La Patra, 1978; Chaitow and Martin, 1988) where it is centred around the notion of whole-person care. In the context of drug training it is important to recognise that the 'whole person' is involved in the learning process and needs to be taken account of in the planning of any learning event. As La Patra points out: 'growing numbers of us are recognising the deep interdependence of body, mind, emotion and spirit, and working towards the good health of all those simultaneously rather than separately' (La Patra, 1978:1).

When planning any training event, then, a holistic approach recognises that an individual is not a fixed static personality but an ever-changing fluid combination of body, mind, emotion, spirit and social elements, and that the following need to be considered:

1 *The physical.* You should make sure that the physical needs of participants are taken care of. To do this *you* have to check out suitable venues. For example, avoid cramped spaces, poorly lit, ventilated or heated rooms and seating that is too hard *or* too comfortable. Are there disabled and crèche facilities available? Make sure that adequate good food is provided and that participants have access to toilet facilities – and know where they are located! A lack of physical activity can lead to a state of low energy levels, fatigue or bodily tension so you should incorporate exercises that involve some physical movement and provide frequent tea/coffee breaks where participants can stand up, stretch or go for a short walk if they want to. Note, however,

that good training can also take place in less than the best physical settings.

2 *The mental.* It is often, and wrongly, assumed that this is the only important part of the person involved in the learning process. Certainly, most people will turn up at a learning event hoping that their mind will be engaged and stimulated, that they will learn things to take away and hopefully put into practice in the workplace. Information can be given to participants by short, lecture-style inputs which can incorporate a question-and-answer session and audio-visual techniques e.g. overheads, slides, videos, to make the presentation more interesting. Make sure you are familiar with audio-visual equipment and feel comfortable using it. You can also give out information in the form of printed handouts, photocopies or other written material. It is important that time should be allowed for adequate discussion of questions and issues raised. Any discussion of issues, however, needs to be grounded in work practice. It is bad training practice for someone to leave a training event without some enhancement of their practical skills.

The key to a successful information-giving session is variety. People can only assimilate so much information in any given time. There needs to be a balance between listening, individual and personal thinking – with space made available for this, perhaps using a short questionnaire – and discussion with other people.

3 *The emotional.* It is important to pay attention to, and be responsive to, the feelings of participants whatever they may be, for example, anger, sadness, fear, joy. This is particularly important when dealing with people who are already working, or are about to work, with intravenous drug users who might be HIV positive or have AIDS. This means, for example, being able to recognise when someone is upset or angry and dealing with it appropriately either at the time or later. The emotional side of working with drug users will be allowed and encouraged to surface in a good training event, and therefore it is essential that the emotional welfare of participants is considered and support mechanisms are built into the event from the beginning.

4 *The spirit.* This means the basic life force or energy that a person has. Participants may need some personal time out or reflection periods during a learning event to replenish their

spirit. Drug workers in particular often arrive at a training event with depleted energy seeking an opportunity to re-energise.

People also need permission to acknowledge their intuitive self. As a trainer you can facilitate this by not denying your own intuitive self and by talking about it openly. Just as workers will act as role models for some drug users, trainers will act as role models for some participants who will watch the way you work, your style, the skills you have and the mistakes you make. You should recognise the effect you can have on participants as a trainer, and the accompanying responsibilities.

Spirit can also refer to a person's spiritual beliefs which are often highlighted and questioned when dealing with training issues around HIV, AIDS and drug use, for example, those that are of a particularly sensitive nature e.g. sex and sexuality, death, dying and bereavement. Although the emotional and the spiritual side of drug work has always been there, HIV and AIDS has brought them more sharply into focus as factors to be considered in the planning of training events.

5 *The social.* It should be remembered that the body, mind, emotions and spirit of a person do not exist in a vacuum but in a social environment. A participant will bring a whole range of past, present and potential social relationships with them on a training event. For example, a drug worker does not work exclusively with drug users but with other drug workers, administrative and managerial staff, people from the community and from other organisations e.g. police, courts, hospitals. This has to be taken account of when planning appropriate training events (see Chapter 5 on groupwork). On the learning event itself people will often learn most from the social relationships they form with other participants during informal breaks and free time. This should be encouraged and can even be formalised into broader networks of mutual support and co-consultancy. Remember, also, that people have personal relationships that they come from and return to. The end of a residential course, for example, can be a shock for people when they have to re-enter the 'real world' and a debriefing session can be useful in helping this process.

The important point to note is that when a person attends a training event they come as a 'whole' person and not just in their worker role portraying their 9.00–5.00 self. *You* should try to be aware of this when you plan, facilitate or lead a learning event. For a more comprehensive account of how the aforementioned approach should influence preparing, designing and leading a training event see the excellent book by Susan Cooper and Cathy Heenan (1980) called *Preparing, Designing, Leading Workshops – A Humanistic Approach.*

The following ideas and principles are derived from their humanistic approach to learning and can be used as a set of guidelines for planning and leading any learning event:

1 *An emphasis on enabling and empowering people.* There are two important factors to keep in mind here:
   (a) Trainers should help people to feel positive about themselves, and the level of knowledge and skills they already have. The learning environment should be co-operative rather than competitive.
   (b) Learning should be oriented to providing participants with a range of information and skills they can *use* in the work setting. What impressions, ideas, information and skills will participants take away that will influence their work with drug users, with other workers, and with individuals and groups in the community?
2 *The use of participants' own resources and experiences.* People will bring a whole range of 'stuff' with them to the learning situation about the particular area or topic they are going to learn. This is particularly true on basic drug courses where people are likely to arrive tightly clutching a range of beliefs, values and attitudes about drugs and drug users that need to be aired and explored at the *beginning* of any course (see Chapter 2 on attitudes). People will also bring relevant work-related experience that can be used in course exercises and should be to their mutual benefit e.g. as case studies, problem-solving exercises.
3 *Participants have a primary responsibility for their own learning.* Learning is a personal and natural process that takes place within the individual. You cannot do it for someone else and they cannot do it for you. You can, however, encourage and motivate people to take responsibility for their own learning by making sure that they play an active role in the learning process. A good trainer:

   should assess students' needs before actually beginning their (workshops) design, and, as much as possible, incorporate these needs into the learning process. In addition to an initial assessment, there should be ongoing feedback between teachers and students that is not only elicited but taken into account.

(Cooper and Heenan, 1980: 4)

Make sure that adequate time is allowed for checking out and processing this feedback from participants during the course.

4 *The trainer is also a learner.* You should, as far as possible, encourage a spirit of 'self-help' so that people will not become over reliant on experts and specialists. The trainer does not have all the answers and learning events should never be allowed to lapse into a 'talking heads' show where the participants are marginalised. 'The open teacher, like a good therapist, establishes rapport and resonance, sensing unspoken needs, conflicts, hopes and fears. Reflecting the learner's autonomy, the teacher spends more time helping to articulate the urgent *questions* than demanding right answers' (Ferguson, 1981: 320). Encourage an atmosphere of shared learning where participants feel free to express their own ideas and feelings. When planning an event you have to decide whether you have the skills and experience to facilitate/teach it yourself or whether you need to hire in someone else to do it. Planning and working with other trainers means you can share and talk about ideas. It also helps you to look after yourself on a training event; you can take time out and will have someone available for support and debriefing. However, note that working with other people can cause problems as well as solve problems (see Chapter 8).

5 *Experiential and participatory learning processes.* People learn best by doing, and a range of exercises, role plays, small-group work and case studies should be devised and included in the design of learning events. Information-giving sessions like lectures or videos, while necessary, should be kept to a minimum. It is what people *do* with the information they are given that is important. Adequate time needs to be allowed for people to question, discuss and process the information while on the event e.g. How do I feel about this information? Is it relevant to my work? How can I use it at work? What more information, if any, do I need? Where do I go from here? The stages of this process are well represented in the learning cycle (Figure 1.3).

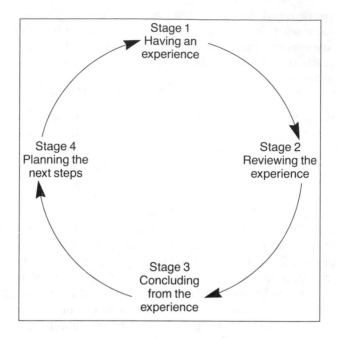

Source: Honey and Mumford, 1986.

Figure 1.3   The learning cycle

As Honey and Mumford (1986) point out, there are several
stages involved in learning from experience and the way we use
these stages will depend on our own individual learning style
(see Appendix 1.1).

6 *Learning involves change.* A person will experience change,
however subtle, whether they are aware of it or not, during a
learning event. Note that change can be about adding something
or taking something away.

> 'Unlearning' is often involved, especially in adulthood. The
> change may be as small as attaching a name to a face or as
> large as making in-depth reorientation in values and self-
> perception – a 'perspective transformation' or 'something of
> a cultural journey'. Fear, anxiety and resistance often ac-
> company and inhibit change.
>
> (Smith, 1984: 36)

Taking account of people's mixed feelings, including fear and anxiety, that are a natural part of the learning process, is essential when planning a course.

7 *Support is essential.* It is important to establish a safe and supportive environment to help people cope with any mixed feelings and to enable them to constructively confront the trainer, other people and, most importantly, themselves. Apart from general support, people can select support groups for themselves for the duration of the course. An exercise for setting up support groups which is relevant for any learning event is included in Chapter 4 on stress management and support systems.

8 *Evaluation is essential.* Evaluation of a learning event gives the trainer information that will be useful for planning and facilitating future events. It can give sponsors information about what participants have learned, how this learning can be effective in practice, and what future training needs are. For some sponsors it will also give relevant information about the cost effectiveness of training and whether they have received 'value for money'. Most importantly, it gives participants a chance to reflect and comment on the course content, structure and administration and an opportunity, at a later date, to explore how useful the course has been for their work practice. There needs, therefore, to be two types of evaluation, depending on course aims and objectives:

(a) *Process evaluation.* All courses will need a feedback sheet that everybody on the course, including facilitators, should complete during the last session. We keep ours simple, use open-ended questions, never give it to people to take away and complete – as they often do not return it! – and always consider the information gained when planning a new course (see Appendix 1.2).

(b) *Outcome evaluation.* Evaluating whether a course has succeeded in its aims of influencing or changing work practice can only be done a few months *after* the course has ended. We build in a follow-up evaluation session on any skills-based course we offer that will usually take place over 1 or 2 days, 3 to 4 months after the course. Examples of this type of evaluation process are given at the end of Chapters 4 and 5.

Remember that training is not a neutral, or value-free, activity. The purpose of this chapter has been to make you think about some of the issues and questions that underlie what training is about and how it is planned and carried out. It is important to be aware of the type of training you are doing and why you are doing it that way. Having read this chapter you can now apply the principles discussed to the following chapters, or any other training.

CHECKLIST

A set of guidelines for doing training

Do you have the right *balance* between training and education in the learning situation?

Have you considered the five *holistic needs* of participants when planning a training event?

Physical
Mental
Emotional
Spiritual
Social

Have you considered the following *principles* based on a humanistic approach to learning?

People need to be enabled and empowered within a supportive learning environment.
People should be encouraged to use their own resources and experiences in the learning situation.
People have a primary responsibility for their own learning.
People learn best through experiential and participatory learning processes.
The trainer is also a learner.
All learning involves change: people have unlimited potential to grow and change and absorb new information.
Support is necessary to cope with change and to allow people to constructively confront the trainer, other people and themselves.
Evaluation is necessary to feedback useful information to trainers, sponsors and participants.

APPENDIX 1.1

Learning styles – general descriptions

There are several different styles that we can use to process any learning experience. Here are general descriptions of four types.

Activists

Activists involve themselves fully and without bias in new experiences. They enjoy the here and now and are happy to be dominated by immediate experiences. They are open-minded, not sceptical, and this tends to make them enthusiastic about anything new. Their philosophy is: 'I'll try anything once.' They tend to act first and consider the consequences afterwards. Their days are filled with activity. They tackle problems by brainstorming. As soon as the excitement from one activity has died down they are busy looking for the next. They tend to thrive on the challenge of new experiences but are bored with implementation and longer term consolidation. They are gregarious people constantly involving themselves with others but, in doing so, they seek to centre all activities around themselves.

Reflectors

Reflectors like to stand back to ponder experiences and observe them from many different perspectives. They collect data, both first hand and from others, and prefer to think about it thoroughly before coming to any conclusion. The thorough collection and analysis of data about experiences and events is what counts so they tend to postpone reaching definitive conclusions for as long as possible. Their philosophy is to be cautious. They are thoughtful people who like to consider all possible angles and implications before making a move. They prefer to take a back seat in meetings and discussions. They enjoy observing other people in action. They listen to others and get the drift of the discussion before making their own points. They tend to adopt a low profile and have a slightly distant, tolerant unruffled air about them. When they act it is part of a wide picture which includes the past as well as the present and others' observations as well as their own.

Theorists

Theorists adapt and integrate observations into complex but logically sound theories. They think problems through in a vertical, step-by-step logical way. They assimilate disparate facts into coherent theories. They tend to be perfectionists who won't rest easy until things are tidy and fit into a rational scheme. They like to analyse and synthesise. They are keen on basic assumptions, principles, theories, models and systems thinking. Their philosophy prizes rationality and logic. 'If it's logical it's good.' Questions they frequently ask are: 'Does it make sense?' 'How does this fit with that?' 'What are the basic assumptions?' They tend to be detached, analytical and dedicated to rational objectivity rather than anything subjective or ambiguous. Their approach to problems is consistently logical. This is their 'mental set' and they rigidly reject anything that doesn't fit with it. They prefer to maximise certainty and feel uncomfortable with subjective judgements, lateral thinking and anything flippant.

Pragmatists

Pragmatists are keen on trying out ideas, theories and techniques to see if they work in practice. They positively search out new ideas and take the first opportunity to experiment with applications. They are the sort of people who return from management courses brimming with new ideas that they want to try out in practice. They like to get on with things and act quickly and confidently on ideas that attract them. They tend to be impatient with ruminating and open-ended discussions. They are essentially practical, down-to-earth people who like making practical decisions and solving problems. They respond to problems and opportunities 'as a challenge'. Their philosophy is: 'There is always a better way' and 'If it *works* it's good.'

(Honey and Mumford, 1986)

To check out which type of learner you are and how you can use learning styles for self-development, see the learning styles questionnaire (LSQ) in 'The manual of learning styles' by Peter Honey and Alan Mumford.

APPENDIX 1.2 FEEDBACK SHEET

Anonymous

Please spend 15–20 minutes considering, then answering, the following questions.

1 What did you like *best* about the course?
2 What did you like *least* about the course?
3 What did you *learn* that will be most useful for your work?
4 What did you think of the administration of the course?
5 What topics would you like included in any follow-up course?
6 Do you have any other comments?

REFERENCES

Abbs, P. (1987) 'Training spells the death of education', *Guardian* 5 January.

Assagioli R. (1971) *Psychosynthesis*, New York: The Viking Press.

Blakeslee, T.R. (1980) *The Right Brain – A New Understanding of the Unconscious Mind and Its Creative Powers*, London: Macmillan.

Brandon, D. (1976) *Zen in the Art of Helping*, London: Routledge & Kegan Paul.

Chaitow, L. and Martin, S. (1988) *A World without AIDS – The Controversial Holistic Health Plan*, Wellingborough: Thorsons.

Cooper, S. and Heenan, C. (1980) *Preparing, Designing, Leading Workshops – A Humanistic Approach*, New York: Van Nostrand Rheinhold.

Dixon, H. and Gordon P. (1987) *Working with Uncertainty – A Handbook for Those Involved in Training on HIV and AIDS*, London: FPA Education Unit.

England, H. (1986) *Social Work as Art-making Sense for Good Practice*, London: Allen & Unwin.

Ferguson, M. (1981) *The Aquarian Conspiracy – Personal and Social Transformation in the 1980s*, Granada: Paladin.

Honey, P. and Mumford, A. (1986) 1 'The manual of learning styles', 2 'Using your learning styles', 3 'The manual of learning opportunities'. (These 3 manuals are available direct from Dr. Peter Honey, Ardingley House, 10 Linden Avenue, Maidenhead, Berks. SL6 6HB.)

La Patra, J. (1978) *Healing – The Caring Revolution in Holistic Medicine*, New York: McGraw-Hill.

Macdonald, D. (1989) 'Skills or issues? The nature of drug training', *Druglink: The Journal on Drug Misuse in Britain* 4 (1): 9.

Polanyi, M. (1983) *The Tacit Dimension*, Gloucester, Mass.: Peter Smith.

Smith, R. (1984) *Learning How to Learn*, London: Open University Press.

Chapter 2

Attitudes to drugs and drug users

This chapter will look at what all people, irrespective of their personal background or work experience, will bring to the learning situation – their attitudes to drugs and drug users. You do not need to be a drug user, know a drug user personally or work with drug users to have formed a set of attitudes. Saturation media coverage of 'drug problems' over the past decade, for example, has ensured that most people will have quite firm ideas about drugs, drug users, and what should be done about the 'drug problem', however biased, stereotyped or misinformed they may be.

> That attitudes to drug use are so strongly held and often so tenuously tied to facts should be a matter of no small concern. How drugs are seen has an important bearing on how drug takers are perceived. Negative and ill-informed beliefs about drugs can be expected to translate themselves into negative and ill-judged reactions to users.
>
> (Griffiths and Pearson, 1988: 13)

Note that although we are dealing in this chapter with attitudes to drugs and drug users, what is said about *attitudes* applies to other topics e.g. HIV and AIDS, and stress, and should be kept in mind when planning *any* course. Also remember that the attitudes component of a course should not be seen as a one-off session, but as a springboard to enable and encourage people to continually reassess and re-evaluate their attitudes.

WHY IS IT IMPORTANT TO EXAMINE ATTITUDES?

There are several reasons why it is important to include people's attitudes towards drugs and drug users in any drug course, particularly at the beginning:

1 It is a good way for people to become *actively involved* in the learning process from the onset. It enables them to look at their own attitudes and beliefs *before* the trainer introduces ideas and examples that may contradict, challenge or criticise those attitudes and beliefs.
2 It is a good way of testing people's *factual knowledge* and will enable trainers to gauge the standard of drug-related knowledge of any group they are working with.
3 It can begin to *normalise* what may be seen as 'sick', 'deviant' or 'criminal' behaviour. The exercise on p. 27 on dependency, for example, looks at the commonalities, the underlying processes and dynamics, that are shared between the drug user and other people. By breaking down barriers between 'them and us' you can encourage and increase understanding and empathy in people who will be working with, or are already working with, drug users.

> Adherence to the narrow view that addiction is something that relates to illicit drugs only has permitted us to maintain the myth that addicts are different. Only 'they' – an alien, deviant, shiftless, nasty and rather dangerous group – use addictive drugs like heroin, and addiction is someone else's problem.
>
> (Krivanek, 1988: vii)

4 Although attitudes may not be an accurate indicator of actual behaviour, they have implications for potential interventions with drug users and for primary and secondary prevention strategies. Holding particular attitudes will have *real consequences* in the practical world. Take the case of workers in an inner-city area who are doing drug training with people in the local community. They are also trying to negotiate the setting up of a needle exchange for local drug users. On the way to work they see government-sponsored posters on billboards and hoardings next to the local community centre (see Figure 2.1) and ask themselves 'How will the images and messages in these posters affect the attitudes of local people towards drug users? How will this affect what I am trying to do in this community?' Generally, workers' attitudes will determine their approach to

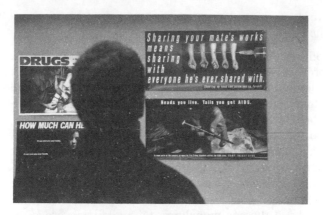

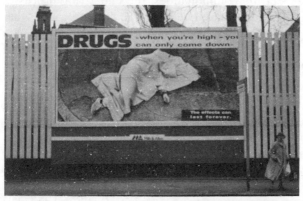

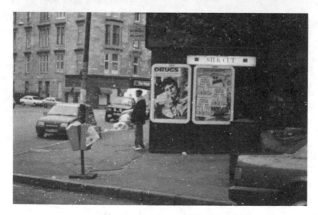

Figure 2.1   Examples of posters

treatment, for example, the differing attitudes of those who believe that abstinence is the only goal of drug treatment in contrast with those who see harm reduction or controlled drug use as viable options.

WHERE DO ATTITUDES COME FROM?

Attitudes are based on sets of beliefs, including stereotypes, that people have about drugs and drug users. They are about feelings and are relatively stable and resistant to change. This means that an attitudes session can be quite emotive and challenging to participants who will have personal investments in maintaining and defending their 'own' attitudes. Remember that people have both private *and* public attitudes. You should aim to create a safe and supportive learning environment where people feel okay about expressing their private attitudes as well as their public ones.

There are 3 components of attitudes that should be kept in mind:

1 They are *descriptive* e.g. 'Drug users look dirty, have long hair and wear earrings.'
2 They are *evaluative* e.g. 'Drug users are sick/bad people.'
3 They are *prescriptive* e.g. 'Drug users should be given long prison sentences.'

There are several exercises you can use to explore these components and the consequences of holding particular stereotypes (see Howe and Wright, 1987: 130, 'Junkie myths – stigma and stereotyping').

The attitudes that people hold are constructed around a complex set of beliefs and values that have been acquired from childhood onwards. They are part of the way that a person experiences and reacts to their world. When discussing the sources of a person's attitudes you need to question how reliable they are and how valid the facts/theories/ideas are on which the attitudes are based. There are four specific sources of attitudes:

1 The mass media and other public information systems
2 The education system
3 Personal contacts like friends, neighbours or relatives
4 Personal experience

> **Exercise**   One way of testing out where a person's infor-
> mation and attitudes about drugs have come from is the
> following:
>
> 1 Ask people to pick a substance they have chosen or
>   decided *not* to use.
> 2 Ask them what information led them to make that decision
>   and from where that information came.

There are several key issues and questions that you can explore,
for example, around the ways that the media presents and portrays
illegal drugs and drug users which in turn informs and helps to
shape people's opinions and attitudes.

1 Does the mass media help to create a 'moral panic':
   (a) by presenting a particular case as universal, e.g. reporting
       that a 13-year-old has died following injecting drugs and
       implying that all teenagers who are injecting drugs and are
       at risk are also likely to die?
   (b) by misinformation being presented as the truth, e.g. that
       experimentation with a drug like heroin leads automatically
       to addiction; that crack is the most addictive substance
       known (ISDD, 1989)?
✓ 2 Does the media over-emphasise and exaggerate the dangers of
     illegal drugs to the exclusion of the danger of alcohol, nicotine,
     over-the-counter and prescription drugs? As Plant points out:

> It is truly a paradox that the greatest drug problems of any
> society invariably relate to those substances which are most
> widely accepted and used. In the British context, this is
> demonstrated by the annual toll of an estimated 100,000
> premature deaths due to tobacco smoking, over 200,000
> drunkenness and drunken-driving convictions, approximately
> 16,000 hospital admissions for alcohol dependence and
> alcohol psychosis and the many thousands of middle-aged
> and elderly people who become dependent upon prescribed
> tranquillisers and sleeping tablets.
>
> (Plant, 1987: 7)

✓ 3 What is the effect of describing drug problems in terms of
     martial imagery, e.g. 'the war on drugs'; 'society's fight against
     the drug pusher' (Trebach, 1987)? How far does this promote
     and support a prohibitionist and law-enforcement stance as the

solution to the drug problem, and therefore the area in which resources should be concentrated?

There is little doubt that the perception that the war on drugs is a failure has spread significantly [in the USA]. It also appears that people are beginning to understand that a war on drugs necessarily breeds violence and corruption.

(Wisotsky, 1988)

4 What is the effect of describing drug problems in terms of medical imagery, e.g. 'drug abuse is an epidemic'; 'drug addiction is a disease'? As Gossop suggests:

in some respects, this view of addiction as a sickness may even be positively harmful. In so far as it perpetuates the myth that the drug addict is a passive and helpless victim of his addiction it contradicts any expectations that the addict can, through his own efforts, learn to live without drugs.

(Gossop 1987: 211)

You can use Figure 2.2 as a framework in which to discuss these, and other, issues and questions. It illustrates several conflicting and overlapping ways of perceiving illegal drug users and therefore the

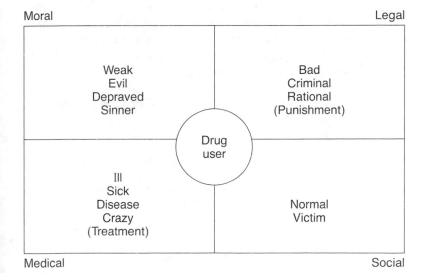

Figure 2.2   Perceptions of illegal drug users

'type' of problem we are dealing with. This is reflected in the various labels that people use to describe drug users, e.g. 'criminal', 'patient', 'client', 'junkie', 'punter'.

There is a story from India that further illustrates Figure 2.2.

> Four blind men were confronted with an elephant. Being blind they obviously did not know what this object was. The first blind man approached the elephant, touched its side, and said, 'This is the wall of a house.' The second blind man approached, touched the elephant's leg and said, 'No it's not, it is a large tree.' At that the third blind man went up to the elephant, touched its trunk, sprang back and exclaimed, 'It's a big snake!' The fourth blind man approached and touched the elephant's tail and said, 'You are all wrong, it's simply a length of rope.' What they all did, of course, was to mistake part of the elephant for the whole elephant.

Similarly with the drug problem, it is all too easy to mistake part of the problem for the whole problem.

Initially, go over the diagram (Figure 2.2) on a board or flipchart and explain what each category means, pointing out the contradictions and complexities:

1 *Moral.* Here the drug user is seen as basically a 'weak' person who may even be acting in a 'depraved' or 'evil' manner, especially if they are selling drugs. This latter view is one quite often favoured by the tabloid press and may engender feelings of shock, anger or moral outrage. You should check with people what their feelings are towards any particular type of drug user, pointing out that it is often not the drug itself that causes this response but the lifestyle of the user or the method by which the drug is taken, particularly intravenous use.

Exercise   To illustrate this point more clearly you can ask participants to close their eyes and imagine a world where the only way to take heroin is to drink it and the only way to take alcohol is to inject it. Which do you think would be seen as the more serious drug problem?

---

2 *Legal.* Here the drug user is perceived as a 'bad' or 'wicked' person engaged in rational criminal activity, involved with dangerous commodities – drugs. Such a person is, by definition,

a criminal who is responsible for their own actions and who may engender fear, mistrust and other such uncomfortable feelings. Punishment, as opposed to treatment, is seen as the solution for dealing with this type of problem. You should be familiar with the debate that suggests criminalisation of a drug may present the user with more problems than the drug itself. In the case of heroin, for example, the user will have to turn to the black market to obtain the drug which may be adulterated with several chemicals causing septicaemia, abscesses or other medical complications. If heroin is in short supply the user may turn to the intravenous use of barbiturates like Tuinal and Seconal and painkillers like Diconal or Temgesic, all more potentially dangerous than heroin itself. Also, if someone uses drugs regularly, they may lie, cheat or steal to obtain the money to pay for blackmarket drugs (Pearson, 1987: 117–47).

3 *Medical.* Here the drug user is seen as someone who is 'sick' or 'ill' (physically and/or mentally) who has a disease, and therefore needs medical treatment. People may feel familiar and more comfortable with this approach because historically there has been a dominance of the medical profession in the treatment and rehabilitation of 'drug addicts'. However, it has its own problems, e.g. how does the 'sick' model reconcile itself with the 'criminal' model? If someone has a disease or is sick, how far can they be held criminally accountable and responsible for their own behaviour? Also, as Bakalaar and Grinspoon point out:

> It becomes part of the definition of this illness that the patients may have no right to decide whether they want treatment for it ... the treatment need not even be for the drug user's own good if drug abuse is regarded as an epidemic.
> (Bakalaar and Grinspoon, 1984: 58)

4 *Social and political.* Here there are several perceptions of the drug user, e.g. as a 'normal' person who has developed a strategy, albeit an illegal and potentially dangerous one, for coping with the strains and pressures of everyday life: as a 'victim' of a particular social environment, for example, someone who lives in a situation characterised by high social, economic or emotional deprivation. There is also the notion of the 'normalisation' of drug taking as an enjoyable recreational human activity within certain social groups. It is ideas like these

that have found expression in the search for a more humane drug policy, e.g. Newsletter of the European Movement for the Normalisation of Drug Policy 1989, the International Anti-prohibitionist League (Arnao, 1988). People holding these, or similar, views may be less judgemental and prejudiced towards drug users and consequently be more able to take into account drug users' perceptions of their own situation when considering intervention strategies.

Exercise
1 After explaining the diagram (see Fig. 2.2) in plenary session ask people which of the perceptions they most agree with and why. You can also ask people how they think the diagram fits in with society's perceptions of other types of drug use.
2 In small groups people can discuss the diagram in relation-ship to their perceptions of particular types of drug user, e.g. a young female intravenous heroin user, a 45-year-old male alcoholic, a recreational cannabis user, someone who has been prescribed valium daily for eight years.

ATTITUDES EXERCISES

We include here some exercises, plus tutors' notes, that can be used to explore people's attitudes to drugs and drug users. Also a list of sources of other exercises (see Appendix 2.1). However, you could consider designing your own exercises or adapting the ones given here to your own needs. What *is* important is that you familiarise yourself with any exercise you use, perhaps testing it out before you use it with a group. It is advisable that anyone using these exercises should have a good working knowledge of drugs and their effects so that they are adequately prepared for any questions or issues raised during discussion.

Exercise A Pie chart – 'the circle of harmfulness' (Figure 2.3) This exercise gives people a chance to explore the origins of their own attitudes to several drugs, both legal and illegal. Do they base their ideas on media information, personal experience of drug taking, or talks with friends and family? It also tests people's factual knowledge about drugs and their effects and what is meant by the notion of a 'harmful' drug.

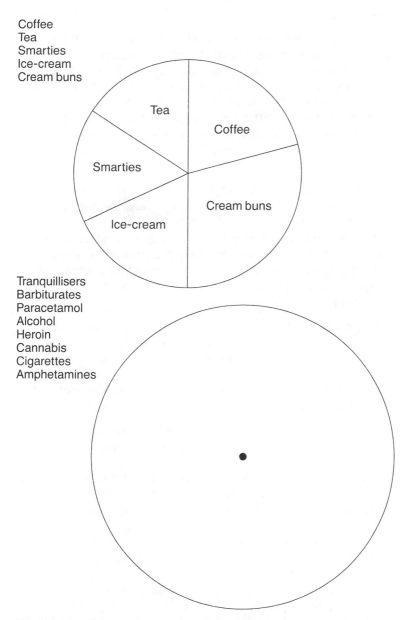

Coffee
Tea
Smarties
Ice-cream
Cream buns

Tranquillisers
Barbiturates
Paracetamol
Alcohol
Heroin
Cannabis
Cigarettes
Amphetamines

Note: Using the substances above, segment the big circle to illustrate your opinion of their relative level of harmfulness. (The small circle is an example.)

Figure 2.3   Pie chart: 'the circle of harmfulness'

Notes for tutors

Each group member should be asked to segment off the large circle as to their perception of the relative harmfulness of each substance listed on the left-hand side. The small circle is given as an example. Ten minutes is the optimum time for completion of the exercise although some people may take a longer/shorter time. Group members, either in pairs or small groups, can then compare and discuss their segments, and the ideas and attitudes on which the segments are based. The following questions can be discussed:

1 Do these ideas/attitudes come from the media, personal experience or that of a close friend or relative, talks with other people, or other sources?
2 What are the consequences of holding these ideas/attitudes? e.g. for intervention with drug users; for prevention strategies.
3 What do people mean by 'harm': is it based on medical, moral, legal or social criteria? Is it harm to the individual, the family, the community or society generally?

Although at first glance this exercise appears simple and straightforward, it is recommended that you only use it if you have a sound knowledge of drugs, their effects, and drug legislation.

For example, do you feel competent to answer the following questions which are just some of those which are commonly asked when using this exercise?

1 What is the 'safe' limit for alcohol? For a man? For a woman?
2 What are tranquillisers? What are their names? What do they do?
3 There is nothing wrong with alcohol, we all like a good drink and it doesn't do us any harm – does it?
4 What are the legal penalties for being in possession of any of these substances?
5 Use of cannabis leads on to other drugs like heroin, doesn't it?
6 I use paracetamol all the time for my migraine – are you saying they are harmful?
7 I've never heard of barbiturates – what are they?
8 How many people die from heroin?
9 What colour is heroin?
10 Have the Government Health Warnings on packets of cigarettes stopped people smoking?

11 What do amphetamines look like?
12 How easy is it to buy any of these substances?
13 Have you used cannabis?
14 What are the dangers of using barbiturates?
15 Are there other more harmful drugs that are not included in this exercise?
16 Would I be better using aspirin than paracetamol?
17 If tranquillisers are prescribed by doctors surely they must be safe?
18 Why are solvents not included in this list?
19 Why is cocaine not included in this list?
20 Is 'crack' the most addictive drug known?

Exercise B Dependency exercise – self-completion question-naire   This exercise enables people to understand the concept of 'dependence' (as well as others such as 'withdrawal' and 'tolerance') by evaluating their own dependent behaviour (see p. 28).

'Dependency' has been chosen rather than the more common, but value-laden and often misused, concept of 'addiction'. Along with the WHO (World Health Organization) we should recognise that the concepts of 'addict' and 'addiction' tend to negatively stigmatise drug users and fail to adequately describe or explain the complexities of being physically and/or psychologically dependent on a drug (WHO *Technical Report Series*, 1964). However, dependency itself is not a completely satisfactory concept to describe and explain the complexities of drug use and you should be aware of the debate around definitions of 'dependency' and 'addiction' (Krivanek, 88: 29–54).

No matter what a person may be dependent on, the processes and stages of all dependencies will have common shared features. Notions about why people take drugs and why they stop taking drugs can be usefully explored using this exercise.

It should be pointed out to participants, however, that there are important unique consequences for people dependent on illegal substances.

Notes for tutors

This exercise should be introduced by suggesting that in order to understand the reasons behind drug users' use and dependency on substances we first need to understand our own dependency on

---

Dependency exercise–self-completion questionnaire Think about one or two things which you use, or have used, on a regular basis and on which you think you are dependent. (These can be legal, illegal or prescribed substances, objects, people, activities – in fact anything you would miss if it no longer existed tomorrow.) Then answer these questions:

1 List your dependency/dependencies.

2 Why do you think you are dependent upon these things? In fact why do you need them, what do they do for you?

3 If you had to give up your dependency tomorrow, how do you think you would feel? Would it be easy of difficult? Would you have withdrawal symptoms?

---

substances, things, activities or people.

You can give some examples of what you mean e.g. a topical TV soap opera, jogging, chocolate, frequent cups of coffee/tea at work, the first cigarette of the day, or a few alcoholic drinks at the end of a busy day.

Try to make your introduction lighthearted as this exercise is meant to be fun.

Ask members of the group to take 10 minutes to fill in their sheets individually, then put them into pairs or threes for 15 minutes to compare notes.

Some people may find this exercise a bit threatening and will need reassurance. You can tell the group that they don't have to identify their own dependency to the others if they don't want to – although most people usually will.

On a flipchart or blackboard you can then list the answers to questions 2 and/or 3 separately, asking for brief responses from each pair/three. Out of this should come substantial material which can be related to the reasons why people use and are dependent upon illegal drugs and the problems they face in giving up drugs.

To do the second part of the exercise i.e. answering question 2, you may want to have available your own list of why people use illegal drugs. The list on p. 29 represents a compilation of reasons given by drug users themselves. This can act as a comparison to the material produced by the exercise as it is likely that there will be many similarities.

Question 3 can be dealt with in the same way but if you're looking for similarities it will tend to be from the point of view of the emotional and psychological withdrawals people experience, e.g. anxiety, unhappiness, pain, loss, etc.

You should also, however, be prepared to answer questions on physical withdrawals.

Good reasons why I take drugs

1 My friends do it
2 It is exciting/fun
3 Tastes good
4 Smells good
5 Feels good
6 Makes me high (life and soul of the party)
7 Relieves boredom
8 Relieves pain
9 Alters my perceptions of reality
10 Cost-effective
11 'Up yours!'
12 It'll never happen to me
13 Instant gratification
14 Sociable
15 Gives me confidence/makes me feel brave
16 Status
17 Pleasure
18 Raises self-esteem
19 Risky
20 Acceptable
21 First/best orgasm I ever had
22 Gives me a feeling of wellbeing
23 Spiritual
24 It's like a career when you're unemployed.

Exercise C   The following exercise can be used as a link between attitudes and the next chapter, 'Drugs and their effects'. The effect of a particular drug on a person can only be gauged by looking *beyond* the drug itself to the *person* using it and the *situation* in which they use it.

Use Figure 2.4, together with the set of questions, to ask people

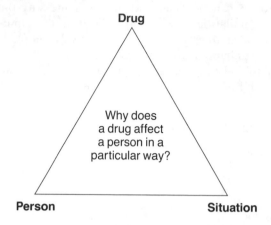

Figure 2.4   Factors influencing the effect of a drug

how alcohol, nicotine or indeed any other drug affects them personally. This will enable you to find out people's attitudes to the very idea of 'drug use' itself.

The following three sets of factors influence the effect that a drug will have. The example given is alcohol, but the model works for any drug, so you could repeat it using the example of the effects of illegal drugs like heroin, cocaine or amphetamines, adapting the questions to suit the specific drug.

1 *Drug*

(a) Amount	How much do you drink?
(b) Strength	What do you drink?
	Does it have a low or high alcohol content?
(c) How you use	Fast or slow drinker?
	Single or mixed drinks?
	Do you drink it or inject it?
(d) Pharmacology	Are there additives or impurities in your drink?
	Is it homemade or shopbought, i.e. quality controlled?

2 *Person*

(a) Personality	How does alcohol affect you? What is your emotional state after drinking? e.g. do you become funny/sad/loud/happy/aggressive, etc.
(b) Personal Characteristics	What is your age? Height? Weight? Sex? General health?
(c) Past Experiences	Are you an experienced drinker? Where and how did you learn to drink? Do you know when to stop? How? What are the signs? Can you 'hold' your drink?
(d) Expectations	What will alcohol do for you? Do you know what to expect? Why?

3 *Situation*

(a) Social surroundings	Do you drink at home or in the pub? Indoors or outdoors?
(b) Other people	Do you feel you have to 'behave' if others are present? How do others react to you when you drink? Do their reactions affect you and your perceptions?
(c) Availability and cost	Would you use less alcohol if it were more expensive? Would you find ways to make it last longer? Would you change if it were more difficult to obtain, or would you make sacrifices to get it?

Now that people have been given time to actively explore their attitudes to drugs and drug users both you and they should have a clearer idea of their current level of knowledge. This will provide invaluable information when you move to the next stage of the learning process about drugs – drugs and their effects.

APPENDIX 2.1

The following is a list of some of the many drug training packs available that include exercises on attitudes. It is not our concern to decide whether any particular training pack is 'good' or 'bad' or 'suitable' or 'unsuitable'. What is important is *how* you use a training pack and adapt its contents to the needs of the group you are working with.

It is the quality of the relationship between trainer and participant that finally determines the usefulness of a training pack:

Dixon, A. and Still, C. (1986) *Working with Drug Users*, London: DHSS/ Optic Nerve.
Howe, B. and Wright, L. (1987) *Drugs: Responding to the Challenge*, London: HEA.
ISDD/TACADE/Life Skills (1986) *Drugwise – Drug Education for Students 14–18*, London: HEC/SHEG.
Jaquet, S. (1989) *Fast Forward Drugs Education Pack*, Edinburgh: SHEG and Youth Clubs Scotland.
Open University (1987) *Drug Use and Misuse*, Milton Keynes: Open University Press.
Pearson, B. (1989) *Multi-disciplinary Drug Training Pack*, Manchester: NWRDTU.

REFERENCES

Arnao, G. (1988) 'International league against prohibition', *The International Journal on Drug Policy* 1 (1):20–1.
Bakalaar, J.B. and Grinspoon, L. (1984) *Drug Control in a Free Society*, New York: Cambridge University Press.
Gossop, M. (1987) *Living with Drugs*, London: Wildwood House.
Griffiths, R. and Pearson, B. (1988) *Working with Drug Users*, London: Wildwood House.
Howe, B. and Wright, L. (1987) *Drugs: Responding to the Challenge*, London: HEA.
Institute for the Study of Drug Dependence (ISDD) (1989) *Crack: A Briefing*, London: ISDD.
Krivanek, J. (1988) *Addiction*, Sydney: Allen & Unwin.
Pearson, G. (1987) *The New Heroin Users*, Oxford: Blackwell.
Plant, M. (1987) *Drugs in Perspective*, London: Hodder & Stoughton.
Trebach, A. (1987) *The Great Drug War*, New York: Macmillan.
Wisotsky, S. (1988) quoted in Wijngaart, G van de (1989) 'Drug abuse research and policy – a Dutch-American debate', *The International Journal on Drug Policy* 1 (3):13.
World Health Organization (1964) 'Expert committee on addiction-producing drugs', *Technical Report Series, 13th Report No. 273*, Geneva: WHO.

Chapter 3

Drugs and their effects

SECTION 1 THE IMPORTANCE OF DRUGS AND THEIR EFFECTS

Before considering the information needed to give people confidence about drugs and their effects, it is recommended that you read Chapter 1 on training methods and approaches. 'Drugs and their Effects', as a session on a course, should not be positioned at the beginning in the belief that this is what the participants want. If this is the case, it says more about the anxiety this session may cause trainers, and illustrates only too well that the model described on p. 4 has not been considered – what is the total package you are trying to offer participants and where does this session fit within that?

Knowing about drugs and their effects does not mean participants will automatically know how to work with drug users. Drugs knowledge must either come *in addition* to existing skills used for working with people, or it must be *an integral part* of a package offering an opportunity to check out participants' attitudes to drugs and drug users, and *to develop* person-centred skills within which to apply that knowledge. If you know how to work with people, then you have a better understanding of working with drug users than if the knowledge you have is based simply on the effects of the drugs they choose to take. This knowledge can, if necessary, be accrued through reading books and useful leaflets as listed in Appendix 3.1. However, it is particularly important to have the opportunity of testing out this knowledge on a course, due to the complex nature of the subject. What can appear complex when studying it alone, can be simplified and checked out in a course environment.

The nature of drugs and their effects is a topic which is constantly changing and it is impossible to teach course participants everything there is to know. It is also difficult as a trainer to keep up to date with new information about different drugs being used, but it is important to be aware of the effects of current 'street' drugs. However, by offering participants a basic grounding in the topic, and how they can enhance their knowledge, you will have equipped them to continue their own learning at a later date. Making this a subject only 'experts' can understand and teach will only serve to prevent people from accepting their own ability to seek out the information for themselves.

Research (Patterson, 1983) suggests that social workers in both the statutory and voluntary sectors, when interviewed to establish the methods of intervention they used working with drug users, were well aware what training was necessary to help them in this area of work. In 1983, as unfortunately is still all too often the case today, there is little education offered on professional qualifying courses into the nature of dependency, nor is there relevant supervision as to how to work in this field. Workers interviewed in the research expressed anxiety about having no perceived knowledge of drugs and their effects, their clients' life styles, nor any control over the chaotic behaviour of their drug-using clients.

Specialised training requested centred round the following topics:

1 Appropriate methods of working with multi-drug users and how current skills could be applied,
2 A practical working knowledge of drugs and their effects,
3 The availability of drugs in society/locally,
4 The drug subculture,
5 'Characteristics' of drug users,
6 Local facilities and resources.

The research showed that workers with a knowledge of drugs and their effects were more confident in their dealings with multidrug users than those without. Often a lack of knowledge would prevent relevant questions being asked about alcohol and other drugs used at an early stage in the assessment process, if indeed any questions were asked at all. This was in spite of more personal questions about financial and emotional matters being asked as a matter of course, which meant that unless the referral and/or the client directly talked of substance use, then it became very difficult for the worker to do so. If not introduced at an early stage in the relationship, harm reduction and general health education were ignored by workers who perceived themselves as having no responsibility for this type of work. Harm reduction, through the discussion of safer use of drugs, is one of the more realistic methods of working used by drug workers, and is an essential component now that HIV is such a major risk (see Chapter 7).

Another conclusion was that the nature or extent of a client's drug use did not seem to affect the method of intervention used by the worker. This indicated not only a lack of knowledge but also an inability to assess how problematic the drug use actually was.

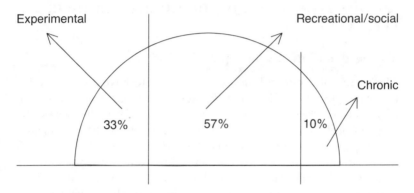

Source: Dixon, 1982a.

Figure 3.1   Prevalence curve of solvent use (North London 1981/2)

Figure 3.1, for example, explains the level of use amongst those young people who had ever tried sniffing or inhaling solvents in an area of North London during 1981/2, and can be equally well applied to other substances which are used illegally. It illustrates three levels of use:

1 *Experimental* – used about 1–6 times, returning to alcohol out of preference, and not using solvents/illegal drugs again.
2 *Recreational/social* – evening and weekend use with friends; this is a social, peer group activity in the same way as alcohol will be for many of you reading this handbook. It is seen as an enjoyable past-time by those involved.
3 *Chronic* – daily, probably more than once per day; often used in isolation from others; with certain types of drugs this level of

use will lead to both physical and psychological dependence; the use of substances will be seen by the user as a solution to the more fundamental problems they have, and may be just the tip of an iceberg.

Identifying the incidence and significance of drug use in someone's life can help to assess whether it is a problem. This assessment can then help you decide on what, if any, should be the subsequent method of intervention. However, without a knowledge of drugs, workers can often lack the confidence to ask the questions which will take them along this useful path.

SECTION 2 THE MYSTIQUE OF 'DRUGS AND THEIR EFFECTS'

You need to demystify the topic

The nature of drugs and their effects seems to have a mystique for many people who work with drug users due in part to the historical approach to treatment and rehabilitation. Over the years the medical profession has dominated the treatment of drug users and, in turn, the knowledge of what effects drugs have. (See pp. 21–3 'Medical' in Chapter 2.) As an increasing number of practitioners with non-medical backgrounds have come into the drug field, they have needed to find ways of accruing enough knowledge to be credible to both drug users *and* doctors, especially psychiatrists.

Often it is easier to learn about the effect of drugs from drug users themselves, although that information should be verified, as some drug users may not clearly understand what the effects of drugs are – particularly when they are mixed. Trying to find the balance between the medical terminology surrounding drugs and the occasionally confused information from drug users has maintained this aura of mystique. Clarifying what is relevant and accurate information can often be a struggle for new workers and volunteers.

The language of the drugs field also plays a part in this mystification process. The perceptions of drug users and what the drug problem is (see pp. 19–24, Chapter 2) have coloured this language, leading to such terms as drug *abuse* or *misuse*. Part of demystifying the words used is to check out with people what they mean when using such terms. Throughout this book people's *drug use* or *drug taking* is referred to rather than their *abuse* or *misuse*. This is based on the belief that words such as abuse and misuse are determined by judgemental attitudes which themselves help to mystify what drug use is all about. Most people who take drugs, be they legal, prescribed or illegal, do not consider themselves to be abusing or misusing them. Abuse or misuse are terms which may relate more to legal or social factors than to harm to the individual (see Chapter 7). These tend to be terms with negative connotations used by those who see themselves as being outside a drug-using subculture. Therefore drug use and drug taking are non-judgemental descriptions and do not force a particular stereotype about drugs or the people who use them onto the participants of any training course. Tackling this demystification process will allow course participants to acknowledge not only the confusion surrounding the language used but also the difficulty of finding their way into this world which is closely guarded on both sides by 'junkies' and 'shrinks'.

The 'expert' debates and disagreements

Another factor which adds to the mystique is that 'drugs and their effects' is not a topic which always offers agreement. Although there are basic principles which can help course participants understand the main effect of a drug (see 'The Basic Guide to Drugs', p. 49), other factors can lead to a wide variety of differing reported experiences of the effects of the same drug. These will be considered later in this chapter on p. 40 'What affects the effect'. However, it is important to draw attention here to one factor which makes it even more problematic for a trainer to give a straight yes or no answer to questions asked about drugs. That is the 'expert' debates about their effects.

Take cannabis as a good example. *The Report of the Expert Group on the Effects of Cannabis Use* (ACMD, 1982) examined a series of commissioned papers on the effects of the use of cannabis and cannabis resin. This was part of the ongoing evidence received by the Advisory Council on the Misuse of Drugs to assist its considerations on implications for future policy (particularly in relation to any recommendations the Council might make about the alleviation of the penalties for unlawful possession of cannabis). As part of the overall conclusions contained in the report the 'expert group' stated:

1 there is insufficient evidence to enable us to reach any un-contestable conclusions as to the effects on the human body of cannabis;
2 but that much of the research undertaken so far has failed to demonstrate positive and significant harmful effects in man attributable solely to the use of cannabis;
3 nevertheless in a number of areas there is evidence to suggest that deleterious effects may result in certain circumstances;
4 there is a continuing need for further research, particularly on the epidemiological characteristics of cannabis use and on the effects of its long-term use by humans;
5 there is evidence to suggest that the therapeutic use of cannabis or of substances derived from it for the treatment of certain

---

Draw the following matrix on a flipchart and ask participants to brainstorm all the drugs they can think of and where they should be placed within the matrix

Socially acceptable	Over-the-counter
Prescribed	Illegal

As participants are shouting out the names of various drugs, disagreement will occur as to where some drugs should go, e.g.

Should cigarettes be placed in the 'socially acceptable' window?
Are magic mushrooms 'illegal'?
Are opiates 'socially acceptable' because they kill pain?
Where should such drugs as diconal and temazepam go?

This allows for the confusion and contradictions to begin to be aired and, as the trainer, you can explain that these disagreements are very much part of the drug field.

Source: Dixon 1979a.

Figure 3.2   The windows or four squares exercise

medical conditions may, after further research, prove to be beneficial.

(ACMD, 1982)

So, given these conclusions, as a trainer what is your response to the question 'Is cannabis harmful?' It would be difficult to offer a hard-and-fast reply and this then adds to the confusion and un-certainty course participants may feel about the subject. Acknowl-edging that uncertainty is another way towards demystifying drugs and their effects, as in certain cases there will be no 'right answer'.

What drugs need to be included?

All types of drugs need to be included when discussing the effects of drugs, that is legal drugs, socially acceptable drugs, illegal drugs, prescribed drugs and drugs which can be bought over the shop counter. Some drugs will fall into more than one of these categories, and this, too, can add to the confusion people may feel. You can use the exercise in Figure 3.2 to highlight this.

This will move you into looking at the breadth of the drugs that need to be considered:

1 Legal drugs, e.g.   alcohol, nicotine and caffeine which is included in tea, coffee, drinking chocolate and soft drinks;

2 Illegal drugs, e.g.   heroin, amphetamines, LSD, ecstacy, cocaine, cannabis and magic mushrooms (under certain circumstances);

3 Prescribed drugs, e.g.   barbiturates like tuinal, nembutal and seconal, tranquil-lisers like valium, ativan and librium, hypnosedatives like temazepam and halcion, pain-killers like diconal, DF118 and temgesic.

Understanding prescribed drugs can be more confusing due to the fact that they can be known by their generic name, brand name and 'street' name, for example:

| Temazepam | Euhypnos, Normison ('jellies'/ 'yellow eggs') |
| Buprenorphine hydrochloride | Temgesic ('tems') |

Sometimes a prescribed drug may be referred to on the street by the name written on the actual tablet, for example:

| Halcion | known as 'Upjohns' |
| 4 Over-the-counter drugs, e.g. | solvents and gases, cough medicines, stomach preparations |

Note. How far do you agree with this categorisation? For example, alcohol, while a legal drug, can also be illegal if consumed under age, and is bought over the counter.

Not all drugs are mentioned here, but this list is included to act as a trigger for your thinking about what drugs may need to be discussed. Rather than give a full list or detailed descriptions as to their effects, it is recommended that you read the literature suggested in Appendix 3.1 to gain a fuller picture of what is useful to know.

What affects the effect

As well as knowing the names of drugs and what category they come under (see The Basic Guide to Drugs, p. 49), it is important that course participants are made aware of the following factors which affect the effect of any drug. The effect may be *physical* and/or *psychological* and, in some cases, may be affected by:

1 *The method of use.*
    Injection – both intravenous and subcutaneous – e.g. of amphetamine, heroin, barbiturates and certain other pre-scribed drugs,
    Smoking – e.g. of nicotine, heroin and cannabis,
    Swallowing – e.g. of cannabis and prescribed drugs,
    Inhalation – e.g. of hydrocarbons found in solvents, fuels and gases like toluene, butane and fluorocarbons,
    Snorting – e.g. of cocaine and amphetamine,
    Sniffing – e.g. of amyl nitrate.
2 *The purity of the drug.*
    'Street drugs' such as heroin and amphetamines are normally 'cut' or adulterated with other substances such as talcum powder or bleach which lowers the purity of the drug,

increases the profit to be made by drug dealers and increases health risks like abscesses and septicaemia. Course participants should recognise that drug users will not normally use 100 per cent pure drug like heroin and that problems can arise from either the substances used to adulterate the drug or, in some cases, the sudden and rare appearance of a more pure drug for sale. Overdoses and possible death can occur from 100 per cent pure heroin.

3   *The mixture of drugs.*
It is normal for many drug users to mix the drugs they take without always being sure of the result. This *polydrug use*, as it is known, is particularly true of illegal drug use, is often chaotic, and usually based on what is available to be taken.
Course participants should be made aware of the possible effects of mixing, for example, heroin and alcohol, or temazepam and alcohol, or a mixture such as heroin and amphetamine.

4   *Physical and psychological disposition.*
The effect of a drug can be affected by certain physical characteristics, for example, the weight, height and general health of a drug user. Increasingly, people with a suppressed immune system due to HIV infection are becoming less able to cope with the effects of drugs. Women are unable to use as much as men because of their lesser height and weight. The menstrual cycle also affects drug use and vice versa. A person's mood can affect the effect of a drug as can any predisposition towards mental illness.

5   *Chemical imbalance.*
The idea that drugs may be used by some to bring about an adjustment in their bodies of an existing chemical imbalance or genetic predisposition is interestingly documented (Wallace, 1988). This has recently been brought to public attention following Bill Werbeniuk, the Canadian snooker player, being given permission to drink a certain amount of lager before playing in tournaments to correct a hereditary chemical imbalance.

6   *Expectations and experience.*
Expectations of the effect of a drug may be based on the information already known about that drug, from friends, films or the written word. These expectations can influence initial use, both negatively and positively. This will be the first experience

which will then colour subsequent use of that drug, and so on.

7 *Social setting and peer-group pressure.*
The feelings induced by using drugs in a warm, comfortable environment will necessarily be different from those resulting from drugs taken up an alley in the pouring rain. Peer-group pressure may dictate that everyone using the same drug, in the same place, at the same time *should* experience the same effects, e.g. groups of solvent users commonly report experiencing similar hallucinations, although this is known not to be true.

8 *Tolerance/cross tolerance.*
The body can develop tolerance to a drug through repeated use which leads to an increased amount of the drug being necessary to achieve the desired effect. This tolerance can also result in cross tolerance with drugs which have a similar effect on the central nervous system, e.g. heroin and alcohol.

9 *Date of last use.*
If someone has not been taking their normal amount of any drug (due to, say, a period of imprisonment or other reason for abstinence), the body's level of tolerance is reduced. This can lead to overdose and possible death if what was their normal amount is suddenly used.

10 *Knowledge of ritual.*
Part of the attraction of drug use often surrounds the rituals involved in the preparation of drugs and the method of use, e.g. preparing the cannabis, rolling the 'joint' and passing it round offers to some a heightened social experience (Becker, 1963). Compare this to offering a packet of cigarettes around.

It is also useful for course participants to have some understanding of:

The availability of drugs.
Particularly those classified as illegal – both locally and nationally.
The 'street names' of drugs.
Particularly those most often used locally.
Cultural preference for drugs and the way they are used.
Do specific ethnic minorities choose to use one drug rather than others? E.g. Rastafarians use marijuana as part of their religious beliefs. Are there drugs which tend to be more popular in one area of the country than in another? For

example, (a) amphetamines are a well-established drug of preference in Scotland, (b) there are differing drinking patterns throughout the country, (c) heroin may be smoked in one area and injected in another (Pearson *et al.*, 1987; Pearson, 1987).

What are course participants' needs?

Professionals often confess that ignorance of drugs and their effects contribute to their unhappiness about working with drug users. It is true that to cope effectively with drug-using clients, one needs to be broadly familiar with the effects of different classes of drugs. However, this does not mean that it is necessary to commit to memory the entire contents of the British Pharmacopeia.

(Griffiths and Pearson, 1988: 17)

In Chapter 8 entitled 'Training the trainers', consideration of establishing at an early stage what participants' needs are will be examined. However, before going on to look at how this topic can be taught, it is important to emphasise what tends to be the overall needs of participants from this part of the course.

What should be sought here is a basic grounding in this complex area. There should be ample opportunity for participants to ask questions of both each other and tutors, and this should be encouraged. Finally, participants need to feel able to continue their learning about drugs and their effects when they leave the course, through books and other literature. They should be encouraged and helped to feel confident in their own learning. It is important to recognise that this enhanced knowledge will improve their service to drug users and their families.

SECTION 3 HOW CAN DRUGS AND THEIR EFFECTS BE TAUGHT?

In looking for methods to teach this topic you should take account of the fact that most participants will have had experience of some of the drugs to be considered, certainly those which fall within the range of legal and over-the-counter drugs. The normalisation of drug use becomes even more apparent when you consider the number of participants who will have had experience of prescribed drugs, particularly painkillers and tranquillisers. Add to them those who may also have either experimented with illegal drugs or used those substances on a more regular basis and there is a range of experience which can usefully be turned into knowledge to share with other participants. Participants, having used exercises to look at their own dependencies, should be beginning to acknowledge that they have within their own experience an understanding of the need for drugs in people's lives. It is now the time to help them look at their own experience and knowledge of drugs. For example, given the statistics and allowing for regional variations, at least 35 per cent (OPCS, 1986a) of the course will have had experience of smoking cigarettes, cigars or pipe tobacco, and at least 96 per cent (OPCS, 1986b; 1988) will have had experience of consuming alcohol ... sometimes with unfortunate results and memories!

If you choose to use a self-completion sheet anonymously (see Appendix 3.2, p. 56–7) either at the beginning or at this stage in the course, you may also discover that some people will have had experience of using opiates as painkillers. This is particularly true when working with women who have experience of childbirth or difficult miscarriages. Take this question further and ask participants what their own experience is, or that of their friends and relatives, of using tranquillisers or other sedatives, and you will no doubt be surprised that as many as half of the participants will either have personal experience or will know of someone who has had long-term use of these drugs. For example, official government statistics show that in 1987 there were 25.5 million prescriptions for benzodiazepines given out in Britain (Hansard, 1989). This extends the wealth of knowledge in the group quite dramatically.

As far as illegal drugs are concerned, people tend to fall into two groups when discussing their use and knowledge of these substances, particularly cannabis. For obvious reasons, many people will resist discussing even their experimental use. Fear of possible repercussions at work, and a desire to forget risks taken in younger years, may well inhibit some participants. However, some may have no anxiety about discussing their illegal drug use, and this can be helpful to the total knowledge base within the course as long as this information will be kept confidential and will not go outside the confines of the course. This type of sharing of experiences can help demystify the belief that it is 'other people' or 'those people' and 'not people like us' who use illegal drugs or drugs illegally.

The anonymous self-completion sheet (Dixon, 1979b) already mentioned (see Appendix 3.2, p. 56–7) can be used to give a total picture of the drug-use experience of people on the course. Once participants have completed it, the trainer can collate the results and show them as a graph, either on a flipchart or on an overhead foil. This not only gives participants information about the experience within the course, but also gives the trainer some idea about how much personal knowledge of drugs there is amongst the participants and therefore how much learning *or* unlearning needs to be done.

The main question you have to ask yourself when considering this topic is whether you will use an 'expert' to talk on the subject, or whether you can use your own and the course-participants' resources to examine what they need to know. Do you want to use an information-based method of teaching this topic or a participatory one? They should not be mutually exclusive, but given an holistic approach to learning, you should look for participatory styles, even when using the didactic approach of the 'expert'.

Let us now go on to consider the various ways of learning about drugs and their effects, both information-based and participatory, and to examine the advantages and disadvantages of each approach.

One of the first steps to take is to attempt to discover what it is people need to know, or think they need to know, to make them more confident with this topic.

Exercise 'What I need to know about drugs and their effects'
(Dixon, 1982b)   Brainstorm in a plenary session the participants' answers to the question: 'What do I need to know about drugs and their effects to make me feel better equipped to work with drug users?' Write the answers on flipcharts around the room and refer back to them during the course to ensure these needs are being met.

This session can then be used to develop the flow of the course in line with the participants' identified needs. This is also a useful way of gaining information which you can return to at the end of any training session to establish whether what people wanted to learn has been covered and, if not, what more needs to be done. Remember not to hurry this process and to give participants ample time to check out what they have learned and how they can take that learning further.

The type of questions participants often identify as important are:

1 What are the drugs people use illegally?
2 What do they look like?
3 How are they taken?
4 How much do they cost?
5 How and where do people buy them?
6 How readily available are they?
7 What effects do they have?
8 What are the signs and symptoms to look out for?
9 What are the risks involved in taking them?
10 What lengths will people go to to acquire these drugs?
11 What are the street names of these drugs?

The type of information necessary to answer some of these questions has been outlined in Section 2 p. 39–42. Some exercises which also help tackle the other questions will be given later in this section.

An example of a 1-day course designed around this topic is as follows:

1 The self-completion questionnaire when people first arrive, to be completed anonymously, which you can collate for a general overview displayed graphically in time for the coffee break, whilst the participants are completing the next exercise.
2 The answers to some of the questions already outlined can be sought from the course participants prior to any contribution by an outside expert or yourself.

It can be useful to set participants homework before they arrive on the course which addresses some of the questions previously mentioned. For instance, questions 1–6 and 11 in the list above can be useful questions for participants to start answering before coming on the course. This can be done by sending out a questionnaire beforehand which can be used on the course in this way.

In small groups, participants are asked to illustrate their findings by writing and/or drawing the information on to flipcharts. The flipcharts are then placed round the walls of the plenary room in time for coffee when everyone can compare answers and representations.

Another way of using this information is in the form of a game for all participants, although some participants may be unhappy about the use of competitive games. 'The Price Is Right!' (Howe and Wright, 1987) is a good example of such a game which helps participants to think about and learn the financial costs of a variety of legal and illegal drugs in their area. The trainer should make up at least twenty cards with the amount of a different drug written on each, e.g.

Litre bottle of Coca-cola
1 gm of cocaine
1 packet of 20 filter-tipped cigarettes
4 Temgesic tablets
8 oz jar of instant coffee
1 gm of heroin
1 bottle of kaolin and morphine mixture
1 oz of cannabis resin

The trainer places three chairs in a row and invites three participants to 'Come on down, the price is right!' Choosing one card at a time, the trainer reads it out and asks the three participants to guess the correct price. The participant giving the closest answer takes the card and returns to the main group. The trainer then asks for another volunteer to 'Come on Down!' When all the cards have been used, answer sheets with the correct prices per substance should be given to all participants.

3 At this stage it is useful to consider 'wheeling in the expert', yourself or otherwise. However, there may be several pitfalls in this approach. The most obvious experts to ask are the local drug-squad officers. Normally they will give a presentation which will include a chance to see the actual drugs involved, particularly the illegal ones. This goes a long way in satisfying the answers to What do the drugs look like? and seems to give those who have not seen these substances before added confidence. The officer may, for example, light up a piece of cannabis so that participants can smell, as well as see and touch, the substance. The style and level of presentation is dependent on the individual officers, although there is a standard basic briefing that they are likely to use. The important point to realise is that whatever the calibre of the presentation, the experience of drug-squad officers is that primarily drawn from a

legal perspective with a corresponding emphasis on illegal drugs. This will by necessity have moral overtones and may reinforce particular stereotypes. Some officers may recount anecdotal tales of arrests, for example, breaking down doors with sledge hammers. Others may talk sensitively of their experiences and opinions of the effect they have seen drugs have on people's lives. You cannot guarantee what the opinion or style of the specific officer will be, but it is worth saying that they will probably hold similar views, given their legal stance.

You will normally have no control over which drug squad officer will do the presentation, as this is dependent on their availability. It will also be unusual to have a woman officer or a black officer make a presentation, as there are so few of them in the drug squad.

It is useful to link the work done by participants in the previous exercise to this presentation, whoever is the presenter. For example, the drug-squad officer will be able to go into detail about what drugs are available locally, what they look like, how they are taken, how much they cost, how and where people buy them, availability, what lengths people will go to to finance their drug use in relation to criminal activity and also what the street names of the drugs are. Should you wish details of the Misuse of Drugs Act included in this session, you may well find that the drug-squad officer can give the relevant and appropriate information about offences under this and other enforceable drug laws. As far as their comments relating to the effects of drugs are concerned, these can be problematic. Often police officers' experience of drug users is at the time of arrest and other such crises, not always the best time to establish an objective view of the effects drugs have on those who use them. Where possible, a presentation or exercise to balance not only the views of the police but also what is said about the effects of drugs would be useful, particularly if this is given by someone who has first-hand knowledge of working with drug users, or even of using drugs themselves.

When considering a presentation relating to the effects of drugs, a medical or pharmacological expert may also be sought. The majority of doctors and pharmacists may well have a sound knowledge of the 'normal' effects of drugs, but may have little experience of the effects people are either seeking from their drug use, or the adverse effects illegal use of prescribed drugs can create. There is also a risk that medical experts, particularly doctors, will mystify the topic even more by using medical jargon. This is most unhelpful if your main aim is to demystify the topic as much as possible.

As already stated, what you should be seeking is a balanced view which takes account of the specific attitudes of those presenting their opinions. If using such presentations, then it is certainly worth including the views and experience of someone who has had direct experience of drugs themselves, or works directly with drug users. Certainly the latter should be available via drug workers or experienced, knowledgeable volunteers in the drug field. However, if you are not making the presentation yourself, it is advisable to ensure you know the content of any contributor's talk, and their attitudes to drugs, drug users and drug problems. This is true with any speaker, but is particularly important here because of the strong moral overtones and unacknowledged biases held by some 'experts'.

4 Another more participatory way of covering this part of the topic, if you have the basic knowledge about drugs and their effects yourself, is to use the material you already have uncovered within the course membership from previous exercises.

Here is one way of specifically looking at the different categories of drugs and their effects.

Exercise 'The Basic Guide to Drugs and Their Effects'[†] (Barrie and Patterson, 1984)   Start by showing an overhead foil with the following statements about three categories of drugs:

Uppers stimulate the central nervous system
Downers sedate the central nervous system
Hallucinogens alter your perceptions of reality

These groups are chosen because the drugs to be classified in each group all have the same overall effect on the central nervous system. You should include painkillers in the downers' group because initially it is better to keep the categories simple. The meanings of these categories should be expanded upon at the time by using the definitions given in the Institute for the Study of Drug

† On our courses this session is called 'Noddy's Guide to Drugs' to bring a little humour into what can often be perceived as a rather humourless session.

Dependence *Drug Abuse Briefing* (ISDD, 1991). Then, using separate overheads with one definition on each at the top, or using one flipchart sheet for the same purpose, ask participants to shout out what drugs they think should come under each category. This will often produce disagreement amongst the participants, with most debate usually occurring around where such drugs as nicotine, cannabis, heroin and alcohol should go. The ISDD *Drug Abuse Briefing* can be used as a guide for any unresolved disputes.

Whilst working through the three categories, you can take the opportunity to show how most drugs actually have more than one effect (Thorley, 1983), by using Figure 3.3 on an overhead foil or as a handout.

Having shown this, check out with participants whether their personal experiences of these drugs correspond to this chart. If not, in what ways do they differ?

The involvement of the group of participants is important as it again allows people an opportunity to see how much they know, to vocalise that if they so wish, and can also encourage discussion around participants' own experience of drug use. Such questions as

Drug	Upper	Downer	Perceptual change
Amphetamine	+++		
Cocaine	+++		+
Caffeine	++		
Nicotine	++	++	
Benzodiazepines		+++	
Alcohol		+++	
Barbiturates	+	+++	
Chlormethiazole	+	+++	
Heroin	+	+++	+
Diconal	++	+++	++
Cannabis	+	++	++
Solvents	+	++	++
LSD			+++
PCP	+	++	+++

+++ Major effect
++ Moderate effect
+ Slight effect

Source: Thorley, 1983.

Figure 3.3   The multi-effects of drugs

what happens when people mix the drugs they use, what are the withdrawals, both physical and psychological, what are the risks attached to different drugs, what do we mean by tolerance and cross-tolerance can be considered, as can some of the myths which may well present themselves during the interaction with the course participants.

One question which can be a problem to answer is: What are the signs and symptoms of drug use?

It is difficult to give hard-and-fast answers to this, as the signs and symptoms of drug use can be diverse. Also, you must be careful making statements about the signs and symptoms that suggest someone is using drugs, as there may be a number of other reasons why someone may be behaving or looking as they do. The notion of change is important, particularly when talking with parents who are most anxious about this whole area. For example, what are the changes you are noticing in someone's behaviour and are there any other reasons which may account for this? If this question is asked by workers, then it is important to ensure that you cover assessment on the course (Dixon, 1987, Chapters 4 and 5: 42–58; Griffiths and Pearson, 1988, Chapter 9: 68–74; Yates, 1982). This will then help them look carefully at their assessment skills and their ability to ask relevant questions about a person's drug use. In Chapter 6, the idea of examining signs and symptoms of drug use is dealt with, but that is very specifically in relation to a course where participants can test out the reality of this using real people as simulated casualties who may or may not be affected by drugs.

5 If it is important for you to show the participants what drugs look like, then you can make up a slide show for that purpose. Your local drug squad may well have such a slide show which they may allow you to buy, or copy.

Alternatively, they may arrange for slides to be taken of the drugs which they use in their presentations. You may also find useful photographs in magazines or books, but remember to check out copyright first before copying them. Combined with the presentation described in Point 4, p. 49 this can make a useful and informative session. This topic can be a difficult area to teach, and it is important to have lively and interesting presentations, which involve participants, and offer ample time for queries to be discussed with the presenter.

6 Relevant wallcharts and literature which you may wish to display as part of a bookstall or use as handouts are

recommended in Appendix 3.1. Lunchtime can often be a good time for such a bookstall.

All of the above will take at least the morning of a day event, and you may find that it can even run over into the afternoon. It is then worth considering involving the participants in more participatory exercises which will bring together what they have already learned in the morning.

7 Three particular exercises recommended for this purpose are:
  (a) 'The costs and benefits of drugs',
  (b) 'So you think you know about drugs' (ISDD and North West Regional Drugs Training Unit, n.d.),
  (c) 'Give me a hand' (Howe and Wright, 1987).

Exercise A 'The costs and benefits of drugs'   Participants go into small groups of no more than nine people. Each small group is then subdivided into three subgroups, and each one of these three subgroups is allocated a specific drug, e.g. alcohol, heroin, cannabis or cocaine. Each participant is given a copy of the ISDD (1991) *Drug Abuse Briefing*, and each subgroup is asked to read what is said in this about their allotted drug, and to complete a flipchart outlining as clearly as possible the costs and benefits of this drug. Allow a maximum of 30 minutes for this. When completed, each subgroup is asked to teach the rest of their small group the costs and benefits of this specific drug – 10 minutes for each drug. Adequate time should be left for discussion.

This exercise encourages people to assimilate knowledge through reading, and then allows them the opportunity to pass on their learning to others. Participants gain more detailed knowledge about three drugs and are also given added confidence in their ability to teach others about drugs.

Exercise B 'So you think you know about drugs'   This short questionnaire with an answer sheet is published by ISDD and North West Regional Drug Training Unit as a training pack. If used towards the end of a day's course on drugs and their effects, it is usefully included in the following way.

Staying in small groups, each participant is given the questionnaire and asked to complete it individually. They are given the answers to check themselves and can then spend some time sharing with each other how they feel about their improved knowledge. This is a good way to end the work in the small groups.

Exercise C 'Give me a hand!' (Howe and Wright, 1987)   This is a non-competitive card game which allows participants to co-operate together in small groups to find the answers to questions about drugs. It is a useful exercise and will take as much time as the 'Costs and benefits' exercise. Other exercises which can be used in small groups are outlined in the teaching packs mentioned in Appendix 2.1. You may have your own tried-and-tested material. Whatever exercise you choose, it is important that participants have the chance to test out their knowledge, in small groups if possible, after any plenary input.

8 A further chance to study the bookstall is recommended during the teabreak.
9 Finally, participants should be brought back together for any questions still left unanswered.
10 It is important to have a resources list available, which should contain two specific types of information. First, national organisations should be included, e.g. the Institute for the Study of Drug Dependence, the Standing Conference on Drug Abuse, the Scottish Drugs Forum, and what service they offer. Second, there should be information on local facilities, both specialist drug agencies and other agencies which offer help to drug users. This will need to be compiled locally and is worth reviewing regularly in order to keep up with any changes.

Teaching a session about drugs and their effects should follow on from participatory exercises and discussion about participants' attitudes to drug use and drug users. This should facilitate greater learning and awareness of any bias on the part of participants or trainers. Participants should be empowered to continue their own learning:

1 by demystifying this topic and showing that you do not have to be an expert to learn and know about the effects of drugs.
2 by using a balance of didactic input and participatory exercises.

It is also important for trainers to learn that it is possible to teach about drugs and their effects without relying on experts or specialists. This has been emphasised throughout the chapter by:

1 examining the pros and cons of different ways and methods of teaching this topic,

2 encouraging trainers to use course participants' knowledge of drugs,
3 helping trainers to realise that by including all drugs in this session they, too, have 'expert' knowledge to offer.

APPENDIX 3.1 OTHER TEACHING MATERIALS

Banks, A. and Waller, T.A.N. (1988) *Drug Misuse: A Practical Handbook for GPs*, Oxford: Blackwell Scientific Publications in association with ISDD.
Blenheim Project (1988) *Changing Gear: A Book for Women Who Use Drugs Illegally*, London: Blenheim Project.
Blenheim Project (1988) *How to Help: A Practical Guide*, London: Blenheim Project.
Field, T. (1985) *Escaping the Dragon*, London: Unwin.
Institute for the Study of Drug Dependence (1986) *The Misuse of Drugs Act Explained*, London: ISDD.
Institute for the Study of Drug Dependence (1988) *Drugs – What Every Parent Should Know*, London: ISDD and IPC Magazines.
Institute for the Study of Drug Dependence (1988) *Surveys and Statistics on Drugtaking in Britain*, London: ISDD.
Institute for the Study of Drug Dependence (1989) *Drug Misuse Wallchart*, London: ISDD.
Institute for the Study of Drug Dependence (1991) *Drug Misuse – A Basic Briefing*, rev. edn, London: ISDD and DHSS.
Open University, Department of Health and Social Welfare in association with the HEA (1987) *Drug Use and Misuse*, Milton Keynes: Open University.
Prentice, Hilary (1985) *Trouble with Tranquillisers*, London: Release Publications Ltd.
Royal College of Psychiatrists (1987) *Drug Scenes*, London: Gaskell.
Scottish Health Education Group (1988) *Drugs and Young People in Scotland*, 4th edn, Edinburgh: SHEG.
Stewart, T. (1987) *The Heroin Users*, London: Pandora.
Trickett, S. (1986) *Coming off Tranquillisers and Sleeping Pills*, Wellingborough: Thorsons.
Turner, P. and Volans, G. (1987) *Drugs Handbook 1987–88*, London: Macmillan.
Tyler, A. (1988) *Street Drugs*, London: Hodder & Stoughton.

Drug Notes Series:
    No 1 Heroin (1986)
    No 2 LSD (1986)
    No 3 Cannabis (1986)
    No 4 Amphetamines (1987)
    No 5 Cocaine (1987)
    No 6 Solvents (1988)

No 7 Tranquillisers (1989)
No 8 Ecstasy (1989)
No 9 Steroids (1989)
    London: ISDD.

'Drugs – users, effects and abuse wallchart' – produced by the Directorate of Public Affairs, Metropolitan Police, New Scotland Yard.

Women and Drinking
Women and Heroin
Women and Smoking
Women and Stimulants
Women and Tranquillisers
    London: DAWN.

Amphetamines (1978)
Cannabis (1978)
Heroin and Other Opiates (1977)
    London: Release Publications Ltd.

APPENDIX 3.2 SELF-COMPLETION SHEET

This is completely anonymous and will be used primarily to illustrate the variation in normal behaviour. See over.

Frequency of use Please tick the highest number which applies to you.	A sleeping drug e.g. barbiturate	Nicotine (cigarettes, etc.)	A tranquilliser e.g. Valium, Librium	An alcoholic drink	A solvent e.g. glues, nail varnish, etc.	Cannabis/ Mari juana
0. Don't know this drug/no comments						
1. Never in my life						
2. Yes, but not in the last 12 months						
3. Yes, during the last 12 months						
4. Yes, in the last 4 weeks						
5. Yes, during the last 7 days						
6. Yes, during the last 24 hours						
7. Yes, today						

Source: Dixon, 1979b.
Note: *e.g. heroin, morphine, pethidine, omnipon, methadone, diconal.

Figure 3.4   Self-completion sheet

Amphetamine/ Cocaine	Coffee, tea or Coca-Cola	Aspirin or Paracetamol (Panadol)	Magic Mushrooms/ Lysergic acid diethylmide (LSD)	*'Controlled opiate' (a) for pleasure	(b) for pain – including surgery, pre-medical or childbirth

REFERENCES

Advisory Council on the Misuse of Drugs (1982) *Report of the Expert Group on the Effects of Cannabis Use*, London: HMSO.

Barrie, K. and Patterson, V. (1984) 'The Basic Guide to Drugs and Their Effects', unpublished course exercise.

Becker, H.S. (1953) *Becoming a Marijuana User*, included in *Outsiders – Studies in the Sociology of Deviance*, New York: The Free Press, 1963, Chapter 3, pp. 41–58.

Dixon, A. (1979a) *The Windows Exercise* (course exercise), London: National Institute for Social Work Course.

Dixon, A. (1979b) *Self-completion Questionnaire* (course exercise), London: National Institute for Social Work Course.

Dixon, A. (1982a) 'Incidence of solvent use amongst young people in North London', unpublished research.

Dixon, A. (1982b) *What I Need to Know about Drugs and Their Effects* (course exercise), London: National Institute for Social Work Course.

Dixon, A. (1987) *Dealing With Drugs*, London: BBC Publications.

Griffiths, R. and Pearson, B. (1988) *Working With Drug Users*, London: Wildwood House.

Hansard (1989) 150 (1481, Col. 389), 10 April.

Howe, B. and Wright, L. (1987) *Drugs – Responding to the Challenge*, London: HEA.

Institute for the Study of Drug Dependence (1988) *Drug Abuse Briefing*, London: ISDD.

North West Regional Drug Training Unit, Manchester (n.d.) *So You Think You Know About Drugs*, London: ISDD.

Office of Population Census and Surveys (OPCS) (1986a) *General Household Survey*, London: HMSO.

Office of Population Census and Surveys (OPCS) (1986b) Eileen Goddard, *Drinking and Attitudes to Licensing in Scotland*, London: HMSO.

Office of Population Census and Surveys (OPCS) (1988) Eileen Goddard and Clare Ikin, *Drinking in England and Wales in 1987*, London: HMSO.

Patterson, V. (1983) 'The management of multi-drug users in social work practice', unpublished research, University of Edinburgh.

Pearson, G. (1987) *The New Heroin Users*, London: Blackwell, pp. 103–4.

Pearson G., Gilman, M. and McIver, S. (1987) *Young People and Heroin*, London: Gower, Chapter 3, pp. 14–17.

Thorley, A. (1983) 'Drugs and their effects', paper presented at Heriot-Watt Drug School, Edinburgh.

Wallace, J. (1988) 'The relevance to clinical care of recent research in neurobiology', *Journal of Substance Abuse Treatment* 5: 207–17.

Yates, R. (1982) *Recreation or Desperation*, a practical guide to assessing drug problems, Manchester: The Lifeline Project.

Chapter 4

Stress management and support systems

Before outlining one training model for running a 5-day 'Stress-Management and Support-Systems' workshop, it is worthwhile considering several issues and questions, particularly: *Why is stress management and support an increasingly important area for drug workers?*

Stress, or rather the inability to cope with stress, is becoming increasingly recognised as a problem for paid workers and volunteers in the helping and caring professions in general. It can lead to many destructive consequences for individuals and organisations alike. A report on *Stress in the Public Sector*, for example, suggests that the collective effects of stress in education and health and welfare organisations are: 'low worker morale; high sickness level; high absenteeism; high staff turnover and wastage; inefficient and ineffective delivery of services; client damage' (HEA, 1988: 9).

Taken together, these effects are symptomatic of what has been labelled 'staff burnout', a condition that may be more likely to affect drug workers than other types of worker in the helping and caring professions (Bailey, 1985). (Note, however, that people do not, literally, 'burn out'! Although a person may be mentally and/or physically exhausted and unable to function, with adequate rest they will recuperate.) In Holland, for example, drug work is seen as having such a high 'burnout' potential that workers are encouraged to work a 4-day week in recognition that they will need a day to unwind from their work before enjoying their 2-day break. Many drug projects in Holland employ a full-time staff guide, often a psychologist, who has a specific responsibility for the welfare of the staff team as a group and also of its individual members, including volunteers (Majoor, 1986).

What is it about drug work that makes it such a high-risk occupation as far as stress is concerned? First, it is important to realise that many of the sources of stress for drug workers mirror the concerns of other types of worker. On one stress-management course held for a group of sixteen drug workers, for example, the following factors were given as some of the sources of stress in the workplace – dealing with other workers, management committees or administrators; a lack of resources; uncertainties about funding; being a particular type of worker, e.g. project leader, detached or outreach worker; unclear project goals; volume of work; time-management problems; lack of supervision and/or support; being seen as an expert; high expectation of clients; cramped office space; feeling isolated. As well as this, drug workers often work with drug users who consistently take risks that other clients do not, for example, with their health, their freedom and their lives. Clients who at times appear to be 'chaotic' can leave workers feeling deskilled and frustrated causing them anxiety about whether the drug user will overdose, will receive a long prison sentence or, latterly, might be body-positive.

THE EFFECT OF HIV AND AIDS

Having to work with people who may or may not be HIV positive and who may or may not at some uncertain time in the future go on to develop AIDS and die, has enormous potential for compounding the stress level of drug workers. Otherwise competent workers may feel anxious and uncertain about the level of skill they have to meet what are perceived as the new needs of users and may require additional skills training in such areas as coping with the chronically sick, sexuality and safer sex, pregnancy, bereavement, loss, health care and hygiene practices, including advice on injecting. They will also have to cope with the increasing anxiety and stress experienced by users who learn they are body-positive. As one drug worker expressed it:

> It's ironic that you are on the point of helping a user renew his life when he is discovering that he may only have a few years left to live. You're helping him to discover new reasons to live then he dies ... you just feel guilty that you haven't done enough.

There are many other increased day-to-day stresses for workers:

Users with HIV constantly talk to me about their 'symptoms' and I try to reassure them while really being uncertain myself whether their nightsweats are caused by the drugs they are taking, by two blankets and a thick duvet, or are the real symptoms of impending AIDS.

Other workers have voiced their concerns about other pressures: 'I'm having hassles with doctors not wanting to examine a drug user with HIV' and 'The stigma of AIDS affects workers as well as clients; there are greater demands and expectations made on us from outside agencies, committees and organisations that we will solve the problem ... yet there are just not enough resources.'

It is important that workers 'practise what they preach'

Many drug workers are engaged in helping users, particularly those with HIV, to learn about relaxation techniques, exercise schedules, diet and nutrition and other stress-management-related skills. In order to do this effectively and credibly they ideally need to have experienced for themselves what it is like to *practise* these skills. Without this practice it can be difficult, and sometimes dangerous, to pass some of these skills on to other people. We would suggest that unless workers are aware of their own stress patterns and are actively developing positive strategies to cope with stress in their lives, they cannot effectively help drug users to understand and cope with their stress.

One problem in setting up a stress-management workshop is that some people come with the expectation that they will be able to successfully manage their stress after a couple of days' work, that all their problems will then be solved. It needs to be carefully emphasised that successful stress management consists of learning coping skills and strategies that require practice and work over a long period of time. Stress patterns that have taken months or years to develop cannot be eradicated in a few days.

A STRESS-MANAGEMENT AND SUPPORT-SYSTEMS WORKSHOP

From our experience of organising and facilitating several different types of stress-management and support-systems workshop for drug workers, we consider the model presented here to be the optimum way of running such a workshop for a group of 16–24 people.

Aims of the workshop

1 To enable participants to identify sources of stress in the workplace,
2 To gain information about stress, its causes, and central issues in its management,
3 To begin to develop positive skills for coping with stress,
4 To begin to develop personal support systems.

The workshop is in two parts:

Part 1 is a 3-day residential course that meets the aforementioned aims.

Part 2 is a 2-day residential follow-up, 3–4 months later that evaluates how successful the workshop has been in effecting change in the participants' work and life.

Both parts of the workshop are planned to be as stress-free and relaxing as possible. This type of workshop should *never* be held in the participants' workplace and should provide a reasonable amount of free time to allow participants to relax. We learned this lesson from the first experimental workshop in stress management we organised, which was based on the principle of recreating a microcosm of the workplace and its stresses and strains during the workshop. While this afforded participants an immediate opportunity to look at how they dealt with any stress that developed, it also increased people's stress to an unacceptable level.

While any stress workshop should be based on principles of empowerment and self-help as outlined in Chapter 1, stress is a topic where the help of an experienced stress consultant or specialist is essential. This should be someone who is familiar with up-to-date information and research in the field of stress management. This person should also have a range of related *practical* skills which can be offered to workshop participants.

Part 1

In order to find out how participants define, experience and cope with stress and what support systems they have available, it is important to have everyone fill in the questionnaire (see Table

Table 4.1 Stress management and support systems workshop questionnaire

Please take some time to consider and reflect on the following questions before you answer them.[†]
 1 Identify the main sources of stress for *you* in your work situation. Please describe in detail.
 2 How do you respond to this stress? Give both positive coping strategies *and* negative responses where applicable.
 3 What personal skills do you have in stress management?
 4 Identify the main sources of stress for *other workers* in your work situation.
 5 How do they respond to this stress? Give both positive coping strategies *and* negative responses where applicable.
 6 What personal skills do they have in stress management?
 7 What support systems exist within your work setting?
 8 How effective are these support systems? If they are *not* effective state why this is the case.
 9 What support systems do you have outside the work setting?
 10 How effective are these support systems? If they are *not* effective state why this is the case.

Note: [†]Alternative instructions for Method A below. Please spend at least 30 minutes thinking about and completing this questionnaire. Ideally you should discuss the relevant questions with the rest of your staff team.

4.1). There are two methods for doing this:

Method A By sending out the questionnaire to participants 3 weeks before the start of the workshop. This has the advantage of gathering information that can be collated and used by trainers in planning the workshop. It can have the disadvantage that people may not send the questionnaire back in time or forget to bring it to the workshop. A stamped addressed envelope can facilitate this.

Method B By giving out the questionnaire to the participants near the beginning of the workshop. This has the advantage of focusing everyone's attention and offering personal space to consider and reflect on the questions. This should be done before identifying common themes, problems and solutions with other workers in a small-group setting. It can have the disadvantage of providing only a limited time period in which to think about, and complete, the questionnaire.

Table 4.2 is the timetable for Part 1. Each session is numbered and named and then explained in the text. Although it is best to run this workshop on a residential basis you can easily adapt the time-table for a non-residential setting. A residential setting is

Table 4.2 Five-day stress management and support systems residential workshop: part 1 (three days)

	Day 1	*Day 2*	*Day 3*
9.30 a.m.–11.00 a.m.		10.00 a.m. Start	*Session 6* Individual and organisational support
11.00 a.m.–11.30 a.m.	Arrival and registration	*Session 4* The nature of stress and positive coping skills COFFEE	
11.30 a.m.–1.00 p.m.	12.00 p.m.	Continued	Continued
1.00 p.m.–2.00 p.m.	*Session 1* Introduction to workshop and support groups	LUNCH	
2.00 p.m.–3.30 p.m.		Continued	*Session 7* Positive coping skills A self-help approach
3.30 p.m.–4.00 p.m.	*Session 2* Self-completion questionnaire and small groups	TEA	
4.00 p.m.–5.00 p.m.		Continued *Session 5* Support groups meet 5.00 p.m.–6.00 p.m.	*Session 8* (a) Support groups meet (b) Evaluation
6.00 p.m.–7.00 p.m.	Small groups (cont.)	DINNER	
7.00 p.m.–8.30 p.m.	*Session 3*	Free	
8.30 p.m.–9.30 p.m.	Support groups meet		

preferred, however, because it enables people to take time out from their normal everyday life of home and work to explore their stress patterns and how they cope with them. It also ensures continuity without the demands of home and work.

Session 1   Introduction to the workshop and support groups

Introduction

There are several ways of facilitating personal introductions at the beginning of *any* workshop or course. The following is one such recommended exercise. It is a good 'ice breaker' as it is non-threatening and enables everybody to participate and talk with others from the outset.

Exercise Introduction   Participants should be sitting in a circle. Time: 10 minutes plus.
Instructions to participants: choose the person you feel you know least. You each have 5 minutes to establish the following information about the other person:

1 Name
2 What project they are from
3 What their journey here was like

You will then each have one minute to introduce your partner to the rest of the group.
Instructions for tutors: your role here is one of timekeeper and facilitator of the group. The instructions to participants may be given verbally or in writing. Once the task has been completed you should facilitate each person's introduction of their partner. This part of the exercise will take as many minutes as there are participants on the course.

At this stage in the workshop there is an optional exercise.

Exercise Expectations   Participants should brainstorm the following question for 5–10 minutes.
Write all the answers on a flipchart and ask the participants to keep a more detailed note of their own answer:
What do you expect to get out of the workshop? Imagine that you leave the workshop feeling good. What would you have learned and/or experienced to feel like that?

There are three ways in which this exercise can be used:

1 As a focus for group discussion immediately after the exercise has been completed,
2 As a check at the end of 3 days to enable participants to assess whether their expectations of the workshop have been met,
3 To provide background information about the group's expectations for the specialist who will be leading Day 2 of the workshop.

Support

As this is a stress-management *and* support-systems workshop, it is important for participants not only to discuss support but also to experience a support group for the duration of the workshop. This can enable people to cope better with any difficulties during the workshop by offering a structured support system. They will also gain practical skills and an understanding of a structure that can be used in the work setting. Members of support groups initiated in this way often continue to use them for support after the workshop has finished.

The next exercise (Figure 4.1) for the self-selection of support groups can be used at the beginning of *any* workshop or course where support groups are necessary. Before doing the exercise it is useful to give a short lecture on the nature of support. Although support can be a very personal thing for people, it is useful to give out some general information that will stimulate thought and discussion. Participants should also be briefed about the purpose of the exercise, that it is intended to help participants select a support group for themselves which will meet on a number of occasions on a formal basis during the workshop.

This exercise can be quite threatening for some people. As a trainer you should facilitate this process by helping people who become stuck to identify their most likely co-supporters.

Session 2 Self-completion questionnaire and small-group exercise

This session should last for between $2\frac{1}{2}$ and 3 hours with at least one break. The purpose of the session is to enable participants to look at what stress means for them, what the main sources of stress are in the workplace, and how they respond to that stress.

Participants are each given a piece of flipchart paper and given 10 minutes to write down the THREE major aspects of support they are looking for from other course members.

For example:

I am looking for the following:	My support needs are:
(a) Good listeners	(a) Constructive criticism
(b) Sympathetic people	(b) A challenge
(c) A chance to relax	(c) Another woman

They should then hold their flipchart in front of them for others to read (or alternatively make a hole in the top of the paper and pull it over their heads) and walk around reading each other's lists. Sufficient time needs to be allowed for this part of the exercise. Once people have read each other's lists, ask them to negotiate and choose two other people whose answers they identify with most closely to form their support triad.

Figure 4.1   Exercise: self-selection of support groups

This should be done in the following way:

1 Give participants 20–30 minutes to fill in the questionnaire (Table 4.1) on p. 63.
2 Divide the large group into smaller task groups of 4–6 people. These small groups can be either self-directed or facilitated.

The task of the small group is to share and compare their answers to questions 1 to 6, particularly questions 1 and 2.

Ask each small group to try and reach an agreement about what the three main sources of stress are for everybody in that group.

These should be written up on a flipchart, along with a list of the other sources of stress talked about within the group.

Another flipchart should be drawn up giving two parallel lists of answers to question 2 for everybody in the group (see Figure 4.2).

Each group should then bring their two completed flipcharts back to the large group where all the charts can be displayed on the wall. Allow at least 30 minutes for discussion within the large group after people have had time to walk around and study each group's charts.

3 main sources of stress in the work situation	Positive coping strategies	Negative responses

Figure 4.2   Flipcharts for answers to questions 1 and 2 of questionnaire (Table 4.1)

Session 3 Support groups meet

Each support group should meet on its own in separate rooms for at least 1 hour. It is up to each group how it runs itself. This is an integral structured part of the course and therefore groups should meet in the rooms allocated to them for the agreed length of time. This should be emphasised because some groups may try and avoid, or be diverted from, the task, e.g. by agreeing to meet in the pub or going for a walk. It should be stressed to participants that what goes on in the group is confidential.

Session 4 External specialist

The whole of Day 2 is given over to a specialist in stress management. Your role as a trainer on Day 2 is to assist the specialist if necessary, or, become a participant for the day, whichever role will be more constructive.

To ensure continuity you should certainly be present at the workshop and not opt out because you have brought in an external tutor.

How Day 2 will be organised in terms of structure and content should be negotiated in advance of the workshop between yourself and the specialist and will depend to a large extent on their level of knowledge and skills.

For example, here are three areas a specialist could cover:

1 Give a lecture on definitions and issues in stress and stress management using the latest research findings. It is important

that both work-related and personal stress are covered here.

2 Do a practical exercise on time-management and goal-setting.

3 Take the group through a relaxation exercise and then talk about key issues in learning a relaxation skill.

For example here are three orientating concepts for people about to learn any relaxation skill. These can be repeatedly re-emphasised while the skill is being learned.

1 Learning a relaxation skill is like learning any skill – e.g. driving a car, typing, swimming – in that there are several stages you are likely to go through. You learn to walk before you learn to run.
   (a) *Regular practice.* Initially you should 'just do it', regular practice is crucial. Repeat what you have been shown and do not worry if there is not much change or you only enjoy some sessions.
   (b) *General benefits.* Although you should not expect too much too soon, after a week or two of regular practice you are likely to notice some general benefits. You may find you are sleeping a bit better, feeling a bit more relaxed, getting less irritable, and so on.
   (c) *Specific benefits.* As you continue to develop your relax-ation skills, specific problem areas that you are particularly bothered by can start to respond. Just as the snowman in the middle of the lawn may take a long while to melt completely when spring comes even though grass is showing through clearly elsewhere, so, too, particular entrenched problem areas may take longer to show improvement than less entrenched general symptoms of tension.
2 *Attention.* When learning a relaxation skill it is important to get the *balance* right between being focused and attentive on the one hand, and relaxing and releasing on the other. Different types of relaxation techniques will have a different balance.
3 *Applications.* When learning a relaxation skill it is important to be able to apply it in various situations. Students can be chal-lenged by having to apply their skill with a noise in the back-ground or when walking or standing. Ultimately they should practise it moving into episodes that previously stressed them.[†]

---

† These ideas are derived from the lecture given by the stress consultant we use on our course, Dr James Hawkins, Edinburgh.

Session 5 Support groups meet

Use the same instructions as for Session 3.

Session 6 Individual and organisational support

The purpose of this session is to enable participants to focus on questions 7–10 of the questionnaire (Table 4.1, p. 63) – to look at what support systems they have both in the workplace and in their personal life, and how effective these are.

You can structure this in a similar manner to Session 2, by dividing the large group into small task groups of 4–6 people.

The task of each group is to share and compare their answers to the questions and then complete flipcharts as in Figure 4.3 as follows. On a flipchart draw up a list of the support systems members of the group have available to them in the workplace. On a separate flipchart draw up a list of what makes these systems effective *and* what makes them ineffective. This exercise can be replicated, if there is time, for support systems outside the work situation.

Again, as with Session 2, allow at least 30 minutes for discussion within the large group after people have had time to walk around and study each group's charts. At the end of this session allow each participant 15–20 minutes to draw on a flipchart a plan for changing and developing their personal support systems, both inside and outside the workplace over the next 3–4 months. You should collect these flipcharts and retain them for use in Part 2 of

Support systems available at work	Why/How effective	Why/How ineffective

Figure 4.3   Flipcharts for answers to questions 7 and 8 of questionnaire (Table 4.1)

the workshop where people will have an opportunity to examine the changes they have made. It should be emphasised to participants that this is 'homework' so only realistic and achievable goals should be identified on these flipcharts. When completed, the flipcharts should be displayed on the wall and time made available for people to look at them. Make sure participants keep a copy of their flipchart on a piece of paper to take away with them.

Session 7 Positive coping skills – a self-help approach

The purpose of this session, which should have been clarified and explained in Session 1, is to encourage people's confidence and ability in their own personal coping skills. It should also enable them to share these skills with others. Participants will already have had time to think about and prepare themselves for this session by completing Question 3 of the questionnaire on Table 4.1, 'What personal skills do you have in stress management?'

One way of organising the session is to ask for volunteers to lead mini-workshops in their particular skills for the rest of the session (about 1 hour). It should be pointed out to participants that 'coping skills' cover not only relaxation-type techniques, but a range of social and political skills like time management, goal setting, assertiveness, negotiation and communication skills. Depending on the size of the group, mini-workshops could range from one person taking a larger group through a relaxation exercise and discussion to a much smaller group where a person who is skilled in successfully negotiating support systems at work shares this knowledge with one or two other people.

Session 8

Support groups meet

Same instructions as for Session 3, except time is limited to 30 minutes.

Workshop evaluation

This session should prepare participants for Part 2 of the workshop in 3–4 months' time and also allow all participants, including facilitators, time to fill in a workshop feedback sheet:

1 Remind participants that Part 2 of the workshop has the aim of evaluating whether or not Part 1 has been effective in producing change in their life, particularly in the workplace. The flipchart completed in Session 6 (see p. 70) will be used as an exercise for this in Part 2.
2 You should now give participants 5 minutes to write down on a flipchart *one* thing they want to change in their life that would reduce their level of stress before Part 2 of the workshop, e.g. take up a sport, exercise more, learn a relaxation skill, cut down alcohol consumption. Emphasise that they should choose something they feel will be readily achieved.
   Collect the flipcharts, making sure participants keep a copy for themselves. These flipcharts will also be used in Part 2.
3 Hand out the feedback sheet (see Appendix 1.2) allowing 10–15 minutes for completion. Before collecting the sheets you can, as an option, ask participants to share some of their comments with the whole group.
4 What about ending a workshop like this? People will need sufficient time to say goodbye to each other in an appropriate manner because of the level of support they will have offered to

Table 4.3 Five-day stress management and support systems residential workshop: part 2 (two days)

	Day 1	Day 2
9.30 a.m.–11.00 a.m.	Arrival and registration	*Session 5* Support systems (cont.)
11.00 a.m.–11.30 a.m.	COFFEE	COFFEE
11.30 a.m.–1.00 p.m.	*Session 1* Questionnaire and review	*Session 6* Positive coping skills – a self-help approach
1.00 p.m.–2.00 p.m.	LUNCH	LUNCH
2.00 p.m.–3.15 p.m.	*Session 2* Review (cont.)	*Session 7* Future planning exercise
3.15 p.m.–3.45 p.m.	TEA	TEA
3.45 p.m.–5.00 p.m.	*Session 3* Support systems	*Session 8* (a) Support groups meet (b) Feedback
5.00 p.m.–6.00 p.m.	*Session 4* Support groups meet	

each other during the workshop. This should be kept in mind when ending any course, but is particularly important when running residential or longer courses of any kind (See Chapter 8 'Training the trainers').

Part 2

The aim of the second part of the workshop is to enable participants to evaluate how successful Part 1 of the workshop has been in effecting change in their lives. Three to four months seems a realistic period of time to give people an opportunity to incorporate and put into action what they have learned as 'homework'. It gives them enough time to try out the efficacy of any new relaxation or other stress-management skill they choose to learn.

Ideally, this part of the course should be done as a 2-day residential workshop, but if time and resources are limited, then it can be done in one day. Table 4.3 illustrates one possible timetable for a 2-day residential workshop.

Sessions 1 and 2   Questionnaire and review

The core of the evaluation process should be built around the questionnaire (Table 4.4) below. This questionnaire should be used along similar lines to the way the questionnaire (Table 4.1) on p. 63 was used in Session 2 of Part 1 of the workshop.

Table 4.4 Post-stress workshop evaluation questionnaire

Please spend *at least* 20 minutes considering and answering the questions.
1 In what ways has the workshop helped you recognise the origins of stress in your life/work?
2 What have you done since the workshop to incorporate ideas of stress-management and support systems into your life/work? (Please specify in detail.)
   IF NOTHING GO ON TO Q.4.
3 What problems, if any, have you encountered in doing this?
   NOW GO ON TO Q.5.
4 Why have you done nothing? (Please specify in detail)
5 How effective do you think the workshop has been as a mechanism for change *and/or* training for you? In what ways could it have been more effective?

Table 4.5 shows the specimen answers to questions 1–3 on Table 4.4 taken from a stress-management workshop.

Table 4.5 Specimen answers to questions 1–3 on Table 4.4 taken from a stress-management workshop

1 In what ways has the workshop helped you recognise the origins of stress in your life/work?

Time away from work to think about and discuss stress.

Good to 'de-individualise' stress and hear and share others' accounts – find out the common denominators.

Confirmed that physical reactions were the result of stress and not just my imagination.

Made me aware that I work too hard.

The influence of outside factors in my attitude to, and performance in, my work.

By offering alleviation of stress in practical, physical and emotional ways it has helped me locate the origins of it.

Made me aware of the anxiety caused by my immersion in the client-based side of my work.

Made me take a step back and look at the situation.

Difficult, stress seems such an intangible thing.

Made me accept that stress is a normal part of work I need to learn to manage.

2 What have you done since the workshop to incorporate ideas of stress-management and support systems into your life/work?

Tried to initiate support group meetings for the staff team.

Allow myself 'time out' if I need it during working hours.

Using some of the practical ideas gained in the workshop.

Organised regular supervision sessions.

Have tried to slow down and 'listen' to myself a bit more, encouraging other workers to do the same.

I now prioritise and manage time more effectively.

Been more assertive in meeting my own needs, learning to say no.

Taken up running.

Set up a 3-tiered support system within the project.

Started a relaxation group.

3 What problems, if any, have you encountered in doing this?

Other workers are cynical and prefer to 'soldier on' as they have always done.

Difficult to discuss work at home.

Only use relaxation techniques on an *ad hoc* basis – do not have the time or self-discipline to use them regularly.

Fear of rejection.

Lack of energy for physical pursuits.

A request for supervision has been misinterpreted as a statement of my not knowing what I am doing and need directed.

Time management is a problem.
Now have two supervisors with different ideas about what I should be doing.
Now seem to have even less time at home.
Too easy to fall back on my old pattern, much easier to be angry and resentful than positively state my limits.
While management acknowledge the level of stress we work under, there is a reluctance on their part to do anything about it.

Sessions 3 and 5 Support systems

These sessions should also use the questionnaire but focus primarily on the personal support-systems charts that participants completed in Part 1.

Participants should go back into their original small groups and discuss where they have reached with the ideas outlined on the chart. They should each then construct a new chart reflecting this. Both charts should be brought back into the large group and displayed on the wall prior to discussion.

Session 4 Support groups meet

The instructions are the same as those outlined in Part 1, p. 68.

Session 6 Positive coping skills – a self-help approach

The instructions are the same as those outlined in Part 1, p. 71.

Session 7 Future-planning exercise

It is useful to give participants a future-planning exercise that encourages them to set goals for the future and recognises the importance of continued development of stress-management skills.

Exercise goal-planning and prioritising Ask participants to write down the following on a sheet of paper:

1 All goals you would like to accomplish in the next five years. Write down anything that comes to mind (2 minutes).
2 Next, list all the goals you hope to accomplish in the next year (2 minutes).

3 Now, list all the goals you hope to accomplish in the next 3 months (2 minutes).

Participants should now look at all three lists and *prioritise* each goal using the following format:

A-goal = those items you have ranked as being most essential and desirable.
B-goal = those items that could be put off for a while but you still feel are important.
C-goal = those items that could be put off indefinitely with little or no harm.

After you have prioritised each list combine the three lists into one list by including two A items from each of your 5-year, 1-year and 3-month goals. Write these down under the heading 'A-priority goals'.

Now, choose two goals from this list that you can realistically achieve within the next 3 months and draw up a plan for achieving them.

Note. Point out to participants at the beginning of the exercise that goals should be realistic and obtainable, and objectives quantifiable. They should also be flexible in the event that they are blocked by other priorities.

(Adapted from Charlesworth and Nathan, 1988).
This exercise can form the basis for a follow-up day to the workshop. If a follow-up day is not possible, participants, in pairs, can make contracts to contact each other by telephone in 2 months' time to check out whether goals have been reached and what has helped and hindered this process.

Session 8 Support groups meet and feedback

This is as outlined in Part 1 (p. 68).
Feedback sheets should be completed for this part of the workshop as in Part 1, Session 8, p. 72.

At the end of Part 2 of the workshop you can offer the participants a further 1-day non-residential follow-up in 3 or 4 months' time. In fact, the participants may well suggest this themselves. This one day will consolidate the learning of relaxation and other stress-management skills and provide an opportunity for the support groups to meet. Some support groups may already be

Coping with personal stress

A regionally based 8-week day release course on Autogenic Training
(Autogenic Training is a powerful self-help relaxation skill)

Note: Autogenic training has been successfully incorporated as part of a self-help treatment package for people with HIV/AIDS by Dr Kai Kermani in London (Kermani, 1988).

A 2-day residential workshop on 'Insight in Crisis' (run in conjunction with staff from the Bristol Cancer Help Centre)

Note: Staff at the Bristol Cancer Help Centre have been coping with the chronically sick, the terminally ill, death, dying and bereavement for several years, and their skills have direct applicability for those workers with HIV/AIDS clients.

Coping with organisational stress

Team development work with individual drug projects

A 2-day residential workshop on Assertiveness Training

'Working on the Front Line'
A 3-day course in communication skills for administrative and secretarial workers in drug projects

Figure 4.4   Related training events arising from the stress-management workshop

meeting after Part 1 of the workshop, but others may find this logistically impossible. A day like this can be repeated several times if necessary.

Overall, we have found that this 5-day workshop has acted as a way-in to finding out about future training needs of participants and can act as a springboard for setting up other related training events. For example, see Figure 4.4.

APPENDIX 4.1 STRESS MANAGEMENT AND SUPPORT – A FURTHER READING LIST

The following recommended titles are a brief selection from the large number available on stress and related fields.

Albrecht, K. (1979) *Stress and the Manager – Making It Work for You*, New York: Simon & Schuster.
Atkinson, J.M. (1988) *Coping with Stress at Work*, Wellingborough: Thorsons.
Benson H. and Klipper M. (1982) *The Relaxation Response*, Glasgow: Collins.
Bliss, E. (1976) *Getting Things Done*, London: Futura.
Booth, A.L. (1985) *Stressmanship*, London: Severn House.
Charlesworth, E.A. and Nathan, R.G. (1988) *Stress Management – A Comprehensive Guide to Wellness*, London: Corgi.
Davis, M., Eshelman, E. and McKay, M. (1987) *The Relaxation and Stress Reduction Workbook*, Oakland, Calif.: New Harbinger Publications.
Douglass, M. and Douglass, D. (1980) *Manage your Time, Manage your Work, Manage Yourself*, New York: Amacom.
Kirsta, A. (1986) *The Book of Stress Survival – How to Relax and Live Positively*, London: Unwin.
Mason, L.S. (1985) *Guide to Stress Reduction*, Berkeley: Celestial Arts.
Mills, J.W. (1982): *Coping with Stress – A Guide to Living*, New York: Wiley.
Pietroni, P. (1986) *Holistic Living – A Guide to Self-Care*, London: Dent.
Simonton, O.C. (1978) *Getting Well Again*, New York: Bantam.

REFERENCES

Bailey R.D. (1985) *Coping with Stress in Caring*, London: Blackwell.
Charlesworth, E. and Nathan, R. (1988) *Stress Management – A Comprehensive Guide to Your Wellbeing*, London: Corgi.
HEA (1988) *Stress in the Public Sector*, London: HMSO.
Kermani, K.S. (1988) 'Stress, emotions, autogenic training and AIDS: a holistic approach to the management of HIV-infected individuals', *Holistic Medicine*, 2.
Majoor, B. (1986) *The Staff Burnout Syndrome in Drug Treatment Programs*, Rotterdam: Karl Hormann Stichting.

Chapter 5

Groupwork

SECTION 1 WHY GROUPWORK?

Although counselling courses are important for drug workers, there are several reasons why a groupwork course is included here rather than a counselling course.

1 Most workers and volunteers either have counselling skills or are offered training courses in those when they start with drug projects. These counselling courses may well be short introductory events, but there is at least an acceptance and an understanding that some knowledge of how to work with people as counsellors is needed.

2 However, this is not the case with groupwork – possibly because formalised groupwork is used less as a method of intervention than counselling and may be seen as less important.

3 Project leaders, managers and management committees may be unable to offer this type of training because they themselves are not skilled in groupwork practice; compared to counselling, groupwork training is difficult to provide within projects and there may be a reluctance to spend limited training monies on external training courses, not necessarily seen as a priority.

4 It may be that there is a general lack of acknowledgement of the time spent by workers and volunteers with drug-related groups. Much of the daily contact possible to workers with drug users can be through their families, peer groups or other community groups. Most drug workers work in teams, some are managed by management committees, and all have contact with other groups of workers, both inside and outside of the drug field, e.g. police, hospital staff, courts. In spite of this there is a general lack of awareness of how useful a knowledge of group

dynamics can be and the potential this offers for a greater understanding of how to be more effective as a worker.

One of the handouts used on the Groupwork Course briefly outlines some of the problems and questions addressed by groupwork for participants. These are expanded here to stress the importance of this way of working. These are general comments and not specific to either workers in the community or those in residential establishments, but are included to make participants think about the relevance and use of groupwork for them.

Problems and questions

User groups

When using groups as a method of working – with drug users' groups and mixed groups – who should be involved? Should you insist on people being 'straight' or not? Should talk about illegal activities be allowed in the groups? What about confidentiality? How do you cope with problems of alliances : dealing : status : scapegoating : drugs on the premises? Consider the use of language – should drug talk and subculture talk be allowed? Consider the risks if members are intoxicated in activity-based groups.

For what purpose are you running therapeutic groups – personal awareness is fine *but* if people have no '*power*' to change their situation, are you not simply adding to their frustration? What are you doing by creating awareness? What are the *political* and *practical implications*? In educational groups that solely pass on information – can drug users listen *and* learn? If so, what techniques can be used to impart health education ideas? Remember people's literacy level and their ability to sit in groups for any length of time. Using groupwork may be appropriate for those who have opted for residential rehabilitation, but is it suitable for client contact in the community?

Family groups

These groups are usually looking for answers to their perceived family problem – can you apply groupwork theory to family groups? If working with family groups there may be conflict

between you and them as to who the perceived client is. This may
be exacerbated by the extreme emotions members may experience
about drug use within families. Who should be involved? For
example, in certain types of family therapy, grandparents, aunts,
uncles and even pets, are involved! Is it possible for family
members to turn words and emotions into actions? Drug use is a
family experience, not that of an individual – can these groups
really take place without the drug user? If a group is there simply
for support, should you intervene as a worker? Should you allow
yourself to take on the leadership role? Should family groups offer
a 'social work' service? What about confidentiality?

Work groups

1 *Management groups and committees.* Do they have the skills
   and experience to manage? How do they show workers they
   care? Can individuals with separate priorities and interests
   remove their professional/political/community hats and work
   as a team to manage a project?
2 *Staff and volunteer groups.* If you have to work together, it is
   like a marriage or a family with all the related problems – what
   happens when staff members leave or the project suddenly
   grows in size through financial expansion? What about intergroup behaviour problems? Alliances? Where does the
   authority and responsibility lie? How effective and efficient is
   the communication within the project? Are the needs of all staff
   and volunteers communicated directly to management? Is there
   a forum for this? Is it only the project leader who attends
   management-committee meetings?

External agencies

How do project members communicate as a team with external
agencies? How is the project perceived by external agencies? How
do project staff and volunteers view their roles as members of
advisory committees or management groups of other agencies?
How does the project liaise with external agencies like the police,
health centres, etc. where intergroup rivalries and conflicts may
occur? In the case of larger organisations, what is known about the
nature of institutions to give an understanding of how institutions
communicate with each other?

Within these different groups there are other questions for workers to think about relating to their knowledge of groupwork, for example: What are your leadership skills and how are you perceived as a leader? What *do* people 'hear' in groups? What is the real communication in groups – non-verbal and otherwise? What are the 'hidden agendas'? Do people *ever really listen* to each other? How does what happens outside the group affect what goes on inside it? Can people be trusted to keep group matters or family matters confidential? What are the ground rules? Does everyone know what they are and agree with them? What are the repercussions if these ground rules are broken?

This is a handout that is used towards the end of the course, but is printed here to help you think about the relevance and applicability of groupwork to drug workers. Beware of those who 'do' groupwork without an awareness of the underlying theories and dynamics.

SECTION 2 ONE WAY OF DEVELOPING A GROUPWORK COURSE

The model offered here is intended for workers and volunteers with no formal education in groupwork theory and practice, but who are working with groups of drug users and/or their families. *'We assume no theoretical knowledge but hope you have some practical experience.'*

The stated aim of the course

'The primary task of the course will be to help your understanding of what goes on in groups and how to apply that understanding to your work, e.g. its appropriateness or otherwise with drug users and how it can enhance your awareness of the processes around in staff groups, management committees and other work groups.'

As this is a 5-day residential course, the information sent out to participants should include a timetable showing the layout of the 5 days indicating the time they have free.

The introductory session should orientate participants to the course, its structure, aims and objectives and methods of learning, and should establish what their expectations of the course are. The methods of learning throughout the week are (a) experiential, (b) didactic and (c) applied, i.e.:

1 Small groups are established to offer course members a personal experience of what it is like to be a group member.
2 These experiences are discussed in the plenary group and a theoretical framework offered to help make sense of what is happening.
3 Participants are then given the opportunity to review how to apply what they have learned on their return to work.

The full timetable is printed in Appendix 5.1. This course is suitable for up to twenty-four participants, with three group tutors, one of whom should have the role of course director. Two basic groupwork books are given to each person, and articles on groupwork with drug users and their families are available for people to read during the week, or to order (see references p. 99–100).

All sessions should be compulsory. Tutors should meet regularly at the same time as the participants' own support groups (see Chapter 4, p. 68). Tutors can be available at stated times for individual consultancy should anyone wish to use that option. In the introductory session it is stressed that this is a participative workshop and that it is up to the participants how it works; that we will look at the underlying processes which take place in groups using a number of groups for that experience which will offer a framework to take back to work at the end of the course.

Is it really possible to plan an experiential course?

The simple answer to this is no because the material that is used in such a course is that which comes from the participants and by necessity is based on their experiences, previous to or at that very moment. However, it is possible to offer a structure within which these experiences can be shared, based on the principle of offering different types of group experience to course participants, e.g. task group, reflection group and consultancy group. This should allow the flow of the course to enable participants to reflect on these experiences and consider how they can apply them at work.

Contents of course

Task groups

As this is a course which is specifically work-related, it is important to begin in a group which mirrors the workplace, so, for the first afternoon and evening, task groups are used. These groups look at specific tasks where group consensus of opinion is sought and then the process by which this agreement, or otherwise, is reached is examined. Two different exercises are used (for example, see Appendix 5.2 for Exercises 1 and 2) both seeking some type of group consensus. However, during the second exercise a more detailed examination of group processes takes place. This is done in a number of ways, with the tutors acting as facilitators. First, permission is given for the equivalent of a group leader to be chosen if the task group so wants. Second, whilst the group are discussing what their decision should be, the facilitator analyses (see Appendix 5.4 for Verbal Analysis Chart) each individual member's verbal intervention to establish whether they are behaving in one of the following ways – task-oriented; group-maintenance or non-functional. That is, are they wanting to complete the task as their overall priority? Are they more interested in maintaining the wellbeing of the group? Or are they behaving in such a way that they appear to be stopping the group from achieving the task or maintaining its cohesion? Third, individual group members are asked to complete a questionnaire (see Appendix 5.3 for questions for participants) which helps them think about how the group coped with the task; what sort of behaviour helped and hindered the group in making its decision; how satisfied they are in the way the group worked; and finally, how committed they are to the final decision.

This individual feedback coupled with the analysis of the behaviour of each member of the group throughout the decision making is given to participants offering them more concrete information for examining what happened. (Details of how to understand and analyse the Verbal Analysis Chart (see Appendix 5.4) are included in Appendix 5.5.)

Plenary group 1

Each morning the course begins with a plenary session which is a time when people can say what they want about the course content, administration or how they are feeling. Sometimes this is known as 'community'. It can be well used or not, but is a useful way of focusing participants into the day ahead.

Reflection groups

The second part of the course is designed to offer participants a chance to reflect on the processes and dynamics which they experienced in their task groups ... hence, reflection groups. The definition of processes is given as 'movements which tend to make for greater psychic comfort on the part of the members' (Douglas, 1978).

Course tutors' roles change from that of active facilitator, to one of observer, commenting either when asked or when it seems appropriate on what is happening within these reflection groups. The material from the task groups allows participants to apply that experience to what is happening in the reflection groups.

Plenary group 2

It is important to offer a didactic input during this part of the course on 'what goes on in groups', using a theoretical framework to help participants' understanding of group processes. This input can be based on one or several theoretical approaches, e.g. Bion (1959), Rogers (1969), the person-centred approach, Gestalt. This input is specifically placed in the middle of the reflection-group sessions in order that the reflection groups can reconvene with a theoretical framework in mind and see if that helps or hinders their understanding.

Support groups

Throughout these two parts of the course, participants are encouraged to use their support groups to talk about how they feel. This type of experiential groupwork can produce extreme feelings, and it is important that when running such an event there are a variety of support mechanisms available for people to use, i.e. small support triads, individual consultancy and, of course, the informal time spent together where much talking and sharing happens.

At this point in the course, a film can be shown which illustrates some aspects of groups. This should be entertaining as well as informative, and is a useful bridge from the more involved, reflective type of groupwork to that which may be more applicable at work. Examples of such films are: *One Flew Over the Cuckoo's Nest, The Bofors Gun, Lord of the Flies, 12 Just Men.*

Plenary group 3

A didactic session on 'Groups at work' helps participants focus their thinking back to the relevance of groups at work. This session is based on the handout used at the start of this chapter, and there should also be space for discussion around the problems identified. At this stage people may be seeing similarities in their roles at work and their role in the reflection groups. This may cause discomfort, but can be useful to acknowledge as this can then be used as material to work with in the consultancy groups which follow.

Consultancy groups

The Consultancy groups are an opportunity for participants to look more closely at problems they are experiencing in work groups, either with management committees, co-workers, client groups or external agencies, and to receive feedback on these problems from other course members. The role of the group tutors here is simply that of timekeeper, as the group members are the consultants. Each course participant is given 10 minutes to talk about a problem at work in relation to groups, and then receives 20 minutes' feedback from the other group members who have remained silent during the 10-minute input. This feedback should be of a supportive nature and if requested by the consultee, constructive criticism is encouraged. This offers everyone the opportunity to have consultancy from a number of others with varying points of view. It also allows each person space and time to consider how to resolve their problem. Participants are given the chance to be a consultant, to listen and concentrate in a group to what is being said. This improves listening skills, sometimes under-rated as a counselling skill. The time allowed can be varied depending on how much time is allowed for this group on the course. At the end of each consultation, the participant whose problem has been reviewed should be given a chance to comment on the experience. This type of group is based on a notion of co-consultancy which is similar to co-counselling, a well-established peer-group self-help method (Evison and Horobin, 1985).

Application groups

The final group used is one which allows participants to look at how they can apply what they have used on the course to their work setting, i.e. application groups. Again this allows the focus to be the work setting but has moved from considering a problem, as in the consultancy group, to how this experience can be applied. Participants may choose to use the problem identified in the consultancy group session and to consider further how they intend to resolve this when they return to work. For example, if a participant has talked about problems they are experiencing in the work team during the consultancy group, and have identified that they played the same role in the reflection group as they do in their staff team, then they are encouraged to take time in the application group to see how they can make changes which will be to their advantage.

Initially each participant is given time and space to identify what it is about their behaviour in groups they would like to change, what they have learned on the course which will help them work towards this change (or will help them live with that part of their behaviour more easily) and what they intend to do about this on their return to work. A discussion then follows in the groups about what each member hopes to work towards based on their individual thinking. Here the group tutor can facilitate the discussion, and it is particularly useful for participants to remain in their consultancy groups for this exercise so that they can see some progress.

Feedback

The course is then evaluated both individually and together in the plenary session:

> The troughs are painful
> To know your limitations is to know your capabilities
> How to resolve unresolved conflict
> Control – need to let go sometimes

The evaluation of this course has produced the answers you might expect to the question: What did you learn that will be most useful for your work? These are comments about knowledge of group processes; some of the theory behind what they can now see happening in groups; what it is like to be a group member as well as a group leader. However, other valuable learning experiences have been identified such as self-awareness; how to handle difficult group members; identifying and understanding their own role in groups; that their own style of leadership is alright; insight into personal authority and how to use it more effectively; the pain and frustration in groups.

SECTION 3 HOW TO HELP WORKERS EVALUATE THEIR LEARNING

With groupwork as with any other skill it is essential that participants have the chance to review what they have learned and how it is applicable to their practice. Therefore, it is recommended that a series of follow-up days be arranged for this purpose, which may help identify new areas of groupwork learning which may be introduced as ongoing training. The first follow-up should be 3 months after the course and can be for 1 or 2 days.

Model for 1-day follow-up

Prior to participants meeting on this day, a questionnaire (see Follow-up day questionnaire in Appendix 5.6) should be sent out which helps course members think about what they learned; how they have applied that learning; what helped and hindered them; and how they want to use the follow-up day. This questionnaire can then be used to structure the day, the timetable of which is as follows:

Table 5.1 Timetable for a 1-day follow-up

10 a.m.	Arrival and coffee
10.15–10.30 a.m.	Plenary and introduction to the day
10.30–12 noon	Small groups which tutors facilitate as task groups, to look at the answers to the questionnaire, and to identify topics for the plenary discussion
12 noon–1 p.m.	Plenary discussion looking at common themes and other responses to the questionnaire
1–2 p.m.	Lunch
2–2.20 p.m.	Individual work based on the question: *Where do I want to go from here?* (see Appendix 5.7).
2.20–3.30 p.m.	Discussion in small groups to identify further areas of learning both at work and as future courses
3.30–4 p.m.	Tea
4–4.30 p.m.	Plenary session to discuss small group session

The result of this day can be a further follow-up day arranged in 4 months' time as requested by participants, which offers consultation groups in the morning, and, for example, the afternoon session run as a 'taster' looking at the Gestalt approach in groups.

The flow chart in Figure 5.1 illustrates what has developed from the original groupwork course and is given as an example of how a follow-up can not only help participants evaluate their learning but also determine what their future training needs are.

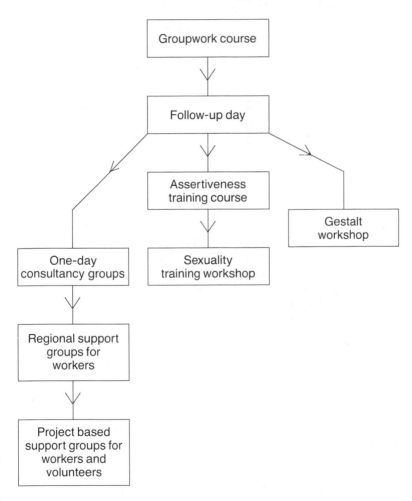

Figure 5.1   A flowchart of related training events arising from the groupwork course

APPENDIX 5.1

Table 5.2 Groupwork course, suggested timetable

	Monday	Tuesday	Wednesday	Thursday	Friday
8.00 a.m.–9.00 a.m.			BREAKFAST		
9.30 a.m.–12.30 p.m. (with break for coffee)	Arrival	Plenary group I leading to reflection groups	1. Plenary review 2. Support groups	1. Plenary group III 'groups at work' 2. Consultation groups	1. Plenary review 2. Application groups 3. Feedback
12.30 p.m.–1.30 p.m.			LUNCH		
2.00 p.m.–5.00 p.m. (with break for tea)	1. Introduction to course 2. Task groups 3. Support groups	1. Reflection groups 2. Plenary group II 'what goes on in groups' 3. Support groups	Free	1. Consultation groups 2. Support groups	Goodbyes and departure
6.00 p.m.–7.00 p.m.			DINNER		
7.30 p.m.–9.00 p.m.	Task groups	Reflection groups	Film	Free	

APPENDIX 5.2

Exercise I The Baron and the Baroness

Tutor's instruction sheet

1 Read the story to the group.
2 Explain that the group must come to an agreement about ascending responsibility for what happened to the baroness.
3 Give the group on a flipchart the cast of characters in order of appearance. These are:
   (a) Baron
   (b) Baroness
   (c) Servants
   (d) Lover
   (e) Gateman
   (f) Boatman
   (g) Friend
4 Do not allow the group to blame external factors such as God or the Government of the day!
5 Ask the group to write down their order of responsibility and give them half an hour to do so.
6 The rest of the time should be devoted to examining the process of their deliberations.

The Baron and the Baroness

This is a story about a Baron and a Baroness. They lived in a castle. Like most castles, this particular one was surrounded by a moat with a drawbridge over it.

One morning the Baron got up and, after having breakfast with his wife, the Baroness, he announced that he was going out for the day. He wanted her to stay at home in the castle and told her that if she went out then something terrible would happen to her.

The Baron then left by his usual means of transport and his wife wandered around for a while wondering what to do with herself. Then, she decided that she was going out. She called for her servants to help her get into her going-out clothes. (As a Baroness she needed people to do this kind of thing for her.) They told her that they had heard what the Baron had said and were very concerned about her decision. She told them that she was making the decisions and to please get on with the job.

She then left the castle and where she went was to a cottage in the wood that surrounded the castle. There she had a meeting with her lover. In fact it was rather more than a meeting and she spent some considerable time before she noticed that the sun was sliding across the sky. She thought to herself, 'Oh, my God, I must get back.' So, she hurriedly got dressed (this time she did it herself). And then hurried back to the castle.

When she got to the castle the drawbridge was up. The gateman was standing there. He told her, 'The drawbridge is up for the night and you cannot get in.'

However, as you will know, all castles have a small door at the back to let people get out if they have to. So, she went round the moat to where the boatman was and asked him if he would take her across the moat to the back door. 'Of course, I'd be glad to take you across', he said, 'but it will cost you money.' As a Baroness, however, she didn't carry money and she explained this to him, and he explained to her that he had a wife and family to keep and that if he didn't see her money then she couldn't get the trip across the moat.

What should she do? She went back to her lover and asked for some money. 'Well, I'm not very sure about that' said the lover. 'This wasn't part of the contract that we had with each other. Our relationship was purely carnal and didn't involve any obligation to become involved in this kind of problem. So I can't give you any money.'

She then went to call on a friend who had a cottage in another part of the woods. She explained the situation to this friend and asked if she could borrow some money. 'Any other day in the year I would have been very happy to give you the money for the boatman', said the friend. 'It just so happens that on this particular day my religious beliefs forbid me to engage in any kind of financial transaction.'

Off she went again to the castle. This time when she reached the front entrance the gateman pulled out his sword and cut off her head.

Who was responsible?

(Adapted from Meade)

Exercise 2 Legislation exercise   You are the Cabinet of the day. All legislation concerning all substances and their use – i.e.

solvents, tobacco, alcohol, illegal, prescribed and other drugs – has been wiped off the Statute Book by the previous Government and it is now your job to create new legislation encompassing all substances, which you believe to be politically acceptable to both yourselves and those who elected you, i.e. your Public! The Prime Minister believes in decision making by consensus within the Cabinet, and also likes Cabinet Ministers to have their own well-thought-out point of view. You have 10 minutes to think about your own views on new legislation – write those down if you want – then there is half-an-hour for the Cabinet to formulate the new legislation. A Prime Minister may be chosen if you wish.

Timing

Tutor reads out the above	5 minutes
Individual work	10 minutes
Group discussion and analysis	30 minutes
Individual question sheet	10 minutes
Group feedback	10 minutes
Tutor feedback based on analysis sheet and discussion	20 minutes

APPENDIX 5.3

Task-group decision-making exercise   Questions for participants

1 How satisfied were you with the way the group worked?
2 How satisfied were you with the way you worked?
3 In what ways, if any, did the group discuss *how* they were going to tackle this task? (i.e. did they identify different ways that it could be approached?)
4 What were the effects of any such discussion?
5 How committed are you to the final decision?
6 In what ways did other members of the group behave which helped the group make a decision?
7 In what ways did other members of the group behave which hindered the group in making a decision?
8 In what ways did you behave which helped the group make a decision?
9 In what ways did you behave which hindered the group in making a decision?
10 How did you feel about doing this exercise?

APPENDIX 5.4

Table 5.3 Verbal analysis chart

Behaviour		John No. of times	Total	Mary No. of times	Total	Robert No. of times	Total	Ellen No. of times	Total	Bill No. of times	Total	Sandra No. of times	Total	Totals
Task oriented	Proposing													
	Seeking information													
	Giving information													
	Summarising													
	Building													
	Testing understanding													
	Encouraging													

Group maintenance — Gatekeeping (Bringing someone in)												
Following (Agreement)												
Realignment												
Open (Self-disclosure)												
Disagreeing (Without a reason)												
Non-functional — Defending/attacking												
Blocking												
Overtalking												
Chatter												

**APPENDIX 5.5 UNDERSTANDING AND ANALYSING
THE VERBAL ANALYSIS CHART ON TABLE 5.3**

The categories of behaviour are defined as follows:

1 *Proposing.* Behaviour which puts forward a new concept, suggestion or course of action.

2 *Seeking information.* Behaviour which seeks facts, opinions or clarification from another individual or individuals.

3 *Giving information.* Behaviour which offers facts, opinions or clarification to other people.

4 *Summarising.* Behaviour which summarises, or otherwise restates in a compact form the content of previous discussions or considerations.

5 *Building.* Behaviour which extends or develops a proposal which has been made by another person.

6 *Testing understanding.* Behaviour which seeks to establish whether or not an earlier contribution has been understood.

7 *Encouraging.* Being warm and friendly to others, praising, encouraging.

8 *Gatekeeping (bringing in).* Trying to make it possible for others to be heard: 'What does Jim think?'

9 *Following.* Accepting someone else's ideas: 'I'll go along with that.'

10 *Realignment.* Changing your mind and switching your support from one proposal to another.

11 *Open.* Non-defensive admission of mistakes or inadequacies that could expose you to ridicule; used to make the group more open.

12 *Disagreeing.* Behaviour involving a conscious and direct declaration of difference of opinion, or criticism of another person's concepts.

13 *Defending/Attacking.* Behaviour which attacks another person or defends one's own behaviour; often involves overt value judgements and contains emotional overtones.

14 *Blocking/difficulty starting.* Behaviour which places difficulty or block in the path of a proposal or concept without offering a reasoned statement of disagreement; such behaviours tend to be rather bold, e.g. 'It won't work' or 'We can't do that.'
Note: Disagreeing, defending/attacking and blocking have much in common; the main differences are that disagreeing involves the use of reason which blocking does not;

defending/attacking involves challenging the person not the idea.

15 *Overtalking (shutting out).* Talking at the same time as others so that two or more people are talking at once.

16 *Chatter.* Talking aimlessly without adding anything to the discussion.

Scoring. This is based on verbal behaviour only. A five-bar-gate system is convenient. Totals can be calculated for both the participants and the behaviour categories. Two of the categories should always be double-counted: 'gatekeeping' (or 'bringing in') is also 'seeking information', although the reverse need not be the case; 'overtalking' (or 'shutting out') will also be one of any of the other categories. It is often useful to have a calculator handy in order to do some sums quickly.

In order to use this scheme it is necessary to have some idea of the crucial behavioural dimensions for a given sort of activity. The activity that will be dealt with here is the *effectiveness of groups.* Rackham and Morgan (1977) have carried out a considerable amount of research on group effectiveness. What they found was that in more effective groups:

1 There was roughly an equal amount of all behaviours apart from gatekeeping, overtalking and chatter.
2 Participants contributed in roughly equal amounts.
3 The ratio of proposing to building was less than 4:1.
4 The ratio of encouraging and following to disagreeing, defending/attacking and blocking was more than 1.5:1.
5 Testing understanding and summarising accounted for more than 10 per cent of total behaviour.
6 The ratio of giving information to seeking information was less than 3:1.
7 Those chairing the group had a ratio of overtalking (shutting out) to gatekeeping (bringing in) of less than 2:1.

This data can be used in training by *comparing* the group being studied with the profile of the effective group as described above.

Behaviour analysis may also be useful for looking at the contribution of *individuals* within the group as well as the group as a whole. One potentially fruitful approach is to look at the type of contribution that an individual makes, paying particular attention to the contribution that he/she makes and both omissions and weaknesses. In order to do this it is useful to group the various separate categories under a series of headings and subheadings. There are no end of possible groupings. Here is one possible example:

1 *Task.*
    (a) *Action.*
        Proposing
        Building
    (b) *Information.*
        Giving information
        Seeking information
    (c) *Criticism.*
        Disagreeing
    (d) *Clarification.*
        Summarising
        Testing understanding
2 *Group maintenance.*
    (a) *Participation.*
        Gatekeeping (bringing in)
    (b) *Support.*
        Encouraging
        Following
    (c) *Openness.*
        Open
        Realignment
3 *Non-Functional.*
        Defending/attacking
        Overtalking (shutting out)

This scheme is essentially a hybrid of Rackham and Morgan (1977) and another classic scheme put forward many years earlier by Bales (1950). The only category defined earlier and not dealt with above is chatter, which may be either non-functional (if it gets in the way) or group maintenance (if it is used as a tension release).

Note. This type of behavioural analysis although useful can be limited. It only gives a static picture, omitting, for example, the sequence of events, the quality of verbal contributions, their impact on the proceedings, feelings, issues and group climate.

This section is adapted from a course handout by Tony Manning (1985) 'Behaviour analysis in interactive skills training'.

References

Bales, R.F. (1950) *Interaction Process Analysis: A Method for the Study of Small Groups,* Addison-Wesley.
Honey, P. (1988) *Improve Your People Skills,* London: Institute of Personnel Management.
Rackham, N. and Morgan, P. (1977) *Behaviour Analysis in Training,* New York: McGraw-Hill.

APPENDIX 5.6 GROUPWORK COURSE FOLLOW-UP-DAY QUESTIONNAIRE

1 Identify at least three significant things you learnt from the course (these can be about yourself, your personal life and your work).
2 Consider in detail how you have applied these since the end of the course (if you have been unable to apply your learning, please go to question 5).
3 What helped you in applying your learning?
4 What hindered you in applying your learning?
5 If you have been unable to do anything, why has this been the case?
6 How useful did you find the books and other teaching materials?
7 How are you going to make use of the follow-up day to consider further work in your project?

APPENDIX 5.7 GROUPWORK COURSE FOLLOW-UP DAY

Participants should spend 20 minutes individually thinking about and answering the following question:
Where do I want to go from here?

REFERENCES

Bion, W.R. (1959) *Experiences in Groups,* London: Tavistock.
Douglas, T. (1978) *Basic Groupwork,* London: Tavistock.
Evison, R. and Horobin, R. (1985) *How to Change Yourself and Your World: A Manual of Co-counselling Theory and Practice,* Sheffield: Co-Counselling Phoenix.
Meade, C. *The Him Book,* Sheffield: Central Library.
Rogers, C. (1969) *Encounter Groups,* Harmondsworth: Penguin.

FURTHER READING

Two suggested books for course participants are:

Douglas, T. (1978) *Basic Groupwork*, London: Tavistock.
Houston, G. (1984), *The Red Book of Groups and How to Lead Them Better*, London: The Rochester Foundation.

OTHER TEACHING MATERIALS

Suggested teaching materials for residential workers:

Collins, T. and Bruce, T. (1984) *Staff Support and Staff Training*, London: Tavistock.
Douglas, T. (1986) *Group Living*, London: Tavistock.
Lennox, D. (1982) *Residential Group Therapy For Children*, London: Tavistock.
Note: The Institute for the Study of Drug Dependence holds a collection of articles on groupwork with drug users. It is recommended that details of these should be obtained.

Chapter 6

Critical incidents and related health problems

SECTION 1 WHAT ARE CRITICAL INCIDENTS AND WHY TRAIN PEOPLE TO HANDLE THEM?

Critical incidents are those events drug workers are likely to worry and fantasise about which fill them with fear and trepidation. Such events leave them feeling helpless and not knowing what to do, for example, incidents such as someone who has overdosed, having to manage an unruly person who is drunk or dealing with a drug user who is fitting due to withdrawals from drugs such as temazepam or barbiturates. These are situations when it is crucial to know not only how to manage what is happening, but also what practical steps if any to take. Such skills as assessment, counselling and communication can be used, but basic first-aid skills can boost the worker's confidence in managing the problem and possibly help to save a life. When faced with incidents of this kind, people's reactions often tend to be negative. They may feel deskilled, paralysed, stressed and intuitively will be in a dilemma about whether to 'fight' or 'flight', i.e. whether to stay and attempt to cope or leave hurriedly. These responses are quite natural. Unfortunately, workers and volunteers in the drug field may well be more at risk of facing drug-induced crises than workers in other parts of the caring professions, and, as trainers, you should therefore be aware of the need to boost their confidence in managing such situations. It is such incidents, in fact, that can lead to an already stressed worker becoming totally worn out.

Practitioners do face critical incidents, even although they may not be a normal or daily occurrence for most drug workers, for example, people phoning to say they have taken a drug overdose, finding people who have overdosed, dealing with countless drunk people or those whose behaviour is aggressive because of their drug use, managing a group of young solvent users in a hostel whilst not realising that you are inhaling the fumes from the hairspray they have used, helping people through LSD trips and solvent-induced hallucinations – to name but a few. A realization that such incidents can be a matter of life or death increases the feeling of responsibility to deal with crises effectively. Attempting to treat someone who is injured when you do not know what you are doing can cause more harm to that person. It is therefore sensible to offer first-aid training to enhance knowledge and boost confidence. This course enables workers and volunteers to have confidence in their own ability to manage critical incidents. It also offers an opportunity to acknowledge that it is normal to feel scared, and that workers need support from others both during and after crises of this kind. Working with intoxicated people or those who are injured or risk injury because of their use of drugs creates stressful emotions in workers. Therefore they need time, space and support to cope with emotions such as fear, panic, anger and helplessness.

SECTION 2 HISTORY OF THE COURSE

This course has been run now since 1985 and is very definitely a training course in the sense that it concentrates on the development of practical skills and having to learn the correct way to do first aid. Participants are trained in the first aid most directly related to drug-induced incidents, and are then given an opportunity to manage simulated incidents using trained casualties, who are members of the British Red Cross.

The course is a co-operative merger between the Drugs Training Project and the Scottish Branch of the British Red Cross. It was created following a request from a social work department to train all their residential, day-care and intermediate-treatment workers in drug awareness, first aid and the management of drug-induced incidents. A young solvent user had died whilst in the care of this local authority, and it was clearly identified that workers needed training in how to deal with such incidents. From the original course which lasts three days, has come an adapted version for those in the drug field lasting two days, which takes account of their existing knowledge of drugs, their effects and related health problems. Both courses will be discussed in greater detail later.

However, before describing the course, it is important to reiterate the *co-operative nature* of this venture. Through working together to run this course, the Drugs Training Project and the Scottish Branch of the British Red Cross attempt to offer a better, more thorough service to those attending the course. By offering a model of good interdisciplinary work, which has positive spin-offs for participants, it is hoped that this may also have an impact on workers' practice, showing that this can lead to an enhanced service to the client.

SECTION 3 COURSE CONTENT

1 Drug awareness
2 Related health problems
3 First aid
4 Managing the incidents
5 Health and Safety at Work

(For the 2- and 3-day timetables, see Appendix 6.1)
Note. Whether this course is run on a 2- or 3-day basis, it is important to ensure that *prior* to managing the practical incidents, *all* participants have knowledge of the following:

1 Drugs and their effects
2 Related health problems and good hygiene practice
3 First aid

Drug awareness

It is important for people to have a certain level of awareness about drugs and their effects before participating in this course. This will necessitate you deciding what level of knowledge your course participants have. If participants have no knowledge of drugs you should offer a one-day Drug Awareness Course, as discussed in Chapter 3, 'Drugs and their effects'.

Related health problems and good hygiene practice

It is important to ensure that participants have information on the following:

1 Septicaemia

2 Abscesses
3 Fitting
4 Hepatitis
5 HIV/AIDS
6 Diet and nutritional problems related to drug use
7 Good hygiene practice for yourself and clients

This can be done in various ways, such as didactic input, handouts and exercises (see 'Good Hygienic Practice' in Appendix 6.2). If you are unsure of what information to give, then seek out specialists who can help you. For example, when discussing 'fitting', an input from the Scottish Epilepsy Association is included in the course. This ensures that participants' knowledge of epilepsy and different types of fits is increased, not just fits related to drug use. Septicaemia – blood poisoning – should be mentioned, and then discussed during the session on poisoning in the first-aid part of the course. Handouts on the basic facts about hepatitis, HIV and AIDS should be given. You may want to consider how much time you give to this area, particularly in relation to HIV/AIDS. Remember that what people need here are the facts to help them deal with possible and actual spillage of body fluids, rather than a complete HIV/AIDS Awareness Course. An opportunity to discuss good hygiene practice in relation to these viruses is important plus handouts covering the important points.

Again it is important to realise the effect caused by giving information on infectious diseases 'blind' to participants. Consider who is on the course and what their existing knowledge is of HIV/AIDS. What are their attitudes to working with people with AIDS, those who are HIV positive or are infected with hepatitis? As a Dutch drug worker said: 'The message of HIV to the client causes shock and that shock reverberates along to the drug worker, causing emotional shock in turn to them. This emotional shock is likely to be passed on to the trainer' (Van Heiningen, 1989).

This course is to help participants cope *practically* with people who may be infected, but you sometimes need to give them space to talk about that *shock* or any other disturbing emotion. One way of accomplishing this is to use the following exercise, which looks at the practicalities of working with hepatitis and HIV. It can be completed as a questionnaire individually, then discussed in groups, bringing hygiene and health-related queries to the large group for a plenary session.

Exercise

1 (a) Can you give an estimate of the incidence of hepatitis and
       HIV amongst your clients?
   (b) On what do you base this estimate?
2 What education/counselling are you giving your clients about
   preventing the spread of these viruses?
3 What personal precautions are you taking?
4 What type of training have you had in this area?
5 What more could you do:
   (a) For your clients
   (b) For your organisation
   (c) For yourself?
6 What are the procedures for preventing the spread of these
   viruses within your project?
   (a) Hepatitis
   (b) HIV
7 What are *your* concerns around hygiene within your place of
   work?

Note. This questionnaire can be adapted to your participants'
needs.

First aid

This is a non-certificate course covering procedures directly
relevant to drug-induced incidents. Procedures covered are:

Theoretical.
Basic principles of first aid
Recovery position
Breathing, bleeding, circulation and resuscitation
Handling and lifting
Poisoning – causes and treatment
Shock
Treatment of wounds and bleeding
Diabetes

Practical.
Recovery position
Choking
Emergency resuscitation
Handling and lifting

Wounds

Bleeding

As with the session on epilepsy (p. 104), you may consider inviting a representative of the British Diabetic Association to present the theoretical information on diabetes. This part of the course *must* be taught by qualified first-aid trainers from one of the recognised first-aid organisations, i.e. the British Red Cross, St. Andrew's Ambulance or St John's Ambulance. Although not essential, it is helpful if the first-aid trainers have an understanding of drugs and their effects and the relevance of first aid to working with drug users. This can easily be achieved by offering such training to those who come to teach first aid, and other members of their organisations.

Managing the incidents

Sixteen simulated incidents have been developed which are an amalgam of ideas of what are considered to be the most useful incidents for course participants to have experience of managing. You may identify more:

1   Drugs overdose in a toilet.
2   Heroin user – gouching.
3   Cannabis user and heroin user together (intoxicated) during a home visit.
4   Known drug user (not intoxicated) with a cut hand.
5   Solvent user (intoxicated) with a cut head.
6   LSD trip – good one or bad one.
7   Amphetamine user experiencing difficult withdrawals.
8   Drunk, obstreperous woman – or man.
9   Self-mutilation with a razor blade – young person.
10 Grand mal epilepsy attack.
11 Diabetic coma.
12 Overconsumption of pills and alcohol resulting in casualty being sick and possible loss of consciousness.
13 Head injury after falling during a fight.
14 Burn on the arm whilst cooking in the kitchen.
15 Heart attack – this was specially developed for community centre staff.
16 Internal injuries after a fight.

Note. Amongst these incidents there are those which are purely drug-induced incidents, drug-induced incidents which necessitate first aid, and first-aid incidents which may or may not be drug-induced. Incidents which are purely drug-induced, e.g. nos 2, 3 and 6, may be a good experience for the drug user, but will necessitate workers having to make decisions about how to manage such events, using their communication skills.

Method

On each course, ten of the incidents are presented, normally in two groups of five on separate days. Participants are put into small groups. As the course is usually run for twenty people, then groups of four are the norm. They are advised to pair up, and to take turns – one pair managing the incident, the other pair observing – then to swap over as they move on to the next incident. This helps the debriefing session after each incident, and gives participants the chance to consider how best to work together, how to share the tasks and how to support each other.

Personnel requirements

At least eleven people will be involved in running the incidents – five casualties, five minders and a timekeeper. The casualties act out the part, the minders look after the casualties ensuring no actual injury occurs, introduce the participants to the incident and take the debriefing session after each group has completed the incident; and the timekeeper keeps the time. This part of the course is strictly timed, and the timekeeper will start all incidents at the same time, finish them all together, then move groups on to the next incident once the debriefing session is completed. A stop watch and whistle are useful for this task. If you have the participants' permission, it is very helpful to video how they manage the incidents. You will thus need someone to be the camera person. Seeing yourself on video making those inevitable mistakes is an excellent way of unwinding and gives everyone permission to laugh about their anxieties and blunders.

Venue requirements

You will need enough space to run the number of incidents you intend to have comfortably. For example, if you run incidents 1, 4, 5, 7 and 10 together you will need a toilet for incident 1, a room for treatment of the injury in incident 4, another room for dealing with incident 5, possibly a corridor and hallway for incident 7 and another room for incident 10. You will also require a plenary room where all participants can congregate before and after the incidents, plus a room for the casualties to make up.

Additional requirements

Hopefully this course will be run jointly with a first-aid organisation. They can then assist you by supplying bandages, dressings, plus gloves to wear whilst bandaging open wounds. You will also need to make the incidents look genuine. Therefore ensure your first-aid casualties supply appropriate make-up, particularly for needle marks and open wounds. Remember aids like syringes, solvents, 'pretend drugs' – whatever it takes to make the scene appear realistic. Think carefully about this beforehand. Remember the film for the video.

Timing

As previously stated, this part of the course must be strictly timed. This gives participants definite boundaries to work within. The following are optimum times for the completion of each incident:

management of incident	7 minutes
debriefing	5 minutes
move to next incident and briefing	3 minutes

Before starting the incidents, it is worth giving people the following instruction:

> This is a chance for you to practise handling real people in simulated situations. Remember that they are real people and should therefore be handled with care. Should anything untoward happen, the minder will stop the incident and you are expected to stop when asked to do so.
> Take this opportunity to consider how you would manage such incidents either by yourself or with another person. Notice your own feelings and emotions. Are you reactive or proactive? How do you behave when you are anxious? If you feel deskilled now,

remember your counselling skills. Communication is an important part of good first aid so remember to communicate with your casualty at all times.

As well as the first aid you have learned, remember to assess the total situation before rushing in to help. What are you dealing with? Who are you dealing with? Where are you? Is it safe? What skills are at your finger tips? (both verbal and non-verbal)?

After dealing with these incidents, consider who you will use for help and support.

Each minder can set up the incident by simply stating the name, if appropriate, of the casualty and what situation the participants are going into, e.g. you have arrived for a meeting at a social work office. You are closing up your project on a Friday afternoon when you hear a noise from an office which should be unoccupied. You are a worker in a residential project and have gone to check that everyone has gone to bed. Setting the scene is sufficient; you do not have to explain what the incident is – the element of surprise makes it more realistic.

At the end of the incidents, you should show the video and have a final debriefing session. Where possible this should include everyone, participants, casualties and minders. Briefing cards on how to deal with the incidents (see Appendix 6.3 for examples) should be available for handouts.

Health and safety at work

You need to address the problems of health and safety at work – what is your and your organisation's responsibility? This is best done after the management of the incidents when specific problems can be discussed, such as how to write up the Accident Book, the contents of the first-aid box, reporting procedures. Do you have a friendly local health care centre or GP to call on for help when hospitalisation is not appropriate? What support can you expect or ask for following such incidents? Do you know how to telephone for an ambulance and the disposal of contaminated material? Basically, how would your project *manage* such incidents? This discussion may best be dealt with in small groups.

SECTION 4 TAKING THIS COURSE INTO THE COMMUNITY

This course is not only taught to staff and volunteers working in drug projects. It was initiated for use with residential, day-centre and intermediate-treatment workers and has been used on many occasions for groups of professionals and volunteers. Venues such as schools, residential homes and community centres have been used – the specific courses for community-centre workers have included stewards, cleaners and canteen workers as participants. These are the front-line staff who are concerned with managing difficult and potentially violent incidents, clearing up spillages of body fluids, like blood and vomit and ensuring good public hygiene in community-centre cafes.

The course has also been run for members of the community – the parents of drug users and ex-users, as well as other members of family-support groups and community volunteers. A modified first-aid course is being tried with current drug users in an attempt to help them deal more effectively with their own and others' drug-induced fits, overdoses and health problems. This is another way of providing education about HIV and AIDS care and prevention for drug users.

The major problems about running such a course are that it takes a great deal of organisation, it is expensive and you need the personnel. This has hindered it becoming as accessible to community groups as it should be. In an attempt to overcome this, the Drugs Training Project and the Scottish Branch of the British Red Cross have produced a video teaching pack (Patterson and Pattison, 1990) of three incidents:

1 Drug overdose in a toilet.
2 Known drug user with a cut hand.
3 Alcohol and pills overdose where casualty is sick and becomes unconscious.

This video teaching pack takes the place of the incidents on this course, and offers participants a chance to see how these can be managed. It should be used in place of 'Managing the incidents', pp. 106–9, on the course layout.

All those participating in the production of the video gave their services voluntarily, in the hope that it would be used widely by community groups and would hopefully save lives.

The *Drug Awareness and First Aid Video Teaching Pack* (£20 plus
p & p) can be purchased from:
Drugs Training Project,
Pathfoot Building,
University of Stirling,
Stirling FK9 4LA,
Scotland, UK

APPENDIX 6.1 DRUG AWARENESS AND FIRST-AID COURSE

Day 1

9.30–10.15	Arrival, welcome and introductions to both the course and to each other.
10.15–10.30	Coffee break.
10.30–11.45	Attitudes to drug use and drug users.
11.45–12.30	Drugs and their effects (presentation).
12.30–1.30	Lunch.
1.30–2.30	Small-group exercise on drugs and their effects.
2.30–3.00	Resources session.
3.00–3.15	Tea break.
3.15–4.30	Basic principles of first aid and resuscitation.
4.30	End of Day 1

Day 2

9.30–10.30	First aid continued (recovery position; control of bleeding).
10.30–10.45	Coffee.
10.45–12.30	First aid continued (control of bleeding, poisoning, diabetes, report writing).
12.30–1.30	Lunch.
1.30–3.00	Practical incidents.
3.00–3.15	Tea.
3.15–3.45	Debriefing of incidents.
3.45–4.30	Handling and lifting.
4.30	End of Day 2.

Day 3

9.30–10.30	Epilepsy input.
10.30–10.45	Coffee.
10.45–12.00	Practical incidents.
12.00–12.30	Debriefing of incidents.
12.30–1.30	Lunch.
1.30–2.30	Hepatitis and HIV input.
2.30–3.15	Review of all practical incidents.
3.15–3.30	Tea.
3.30–4.15	'What can we take back from this course?' – Health and Safety at Work (Small-group exercise).
4.15–4.45	Feedback
4.45	End of course.

APPENDIX 6.2 GOOD HYGIENIC PRACTICE

There are a variety of infections related to drug use. Two of the more commonly associated conditions are the hepatitis B virus and the human immuno-deficiency virus (HIV). Outlined below are good hygienic practices which are relevant to this course and which can be used as a handout. It is important to remember that good hygienic practice is part of everyday living and is the responsibility of us all.

Table 6.1 Good hygienic practice in relation to hepatitis B and HIV

Hepatitis B		HIV	
Method of transmission	*Good hygienic practice*	*Method of transmission*	*Good hygienic practice*
1 Blood-to-blood		1 Blood-to-blood	
(a) Needles and syringes	(a) Where possible do not share needles and syringes (for further information on cleaning injection equipment, see *The Cleaning of Injecting Equipment* published by The Department of Health and The Standing Conference on Drug Abuse).	(a) Needles and syringes	(a) Where possible do not share needles and syringes (for further information on cleaning injection equipment, see Hepatitis B, 1(a)).
(b) Cuts and wounds (on other people)	(b) Where possible, use Latex rubber gloves before handling an open cut or wound. If, however, these are not available, minimise	(b) Cuts and wounds (on other people)	(b) Where possible, use Latex rubber gloves before handling an open cut or wound. If, however, these are not available, minimise

Table 6.1 continued

Hepatitis B		HIV	
Method of transmission	*Good hygienic practice*	*Method of transmission*	*Good hygienic practice*
	contact with blood using available materials. Remember to wash your hands immediately with hot water and soap after dealing with this situation.		contact with blood using available materials. Remember to wash your hands immediately with hot water and soap after dealing with this situation.
(c) Cuts and wounds (on self)	(c) Always check your hands for minor abrasions and cuts. These should be covered using an adhesive dressing.	(c) Cuts and wounds (on self)	(c) Always check your hands for minor abrasions and cuts. These should be covered using an adhesive dressing.
(d) Spillage on clothes	(d) If the spillage is *major*, where possible, burn contaminated clothing. Alternatively, bag in two polythene bags securely labelled CONTAMINATED CLOTHING and	(d) Spillage on clothes	(d) If the spillage is *major*, where possible, burn contaminated clothing. Alternatively, bag in two polythene bags securely labelled CONTAMINATED CLOTHING and

arrange disposal by your local Council. If the spillage is *minor*, wash in as high a temperature as the fabric will allow in a washing machine. In both cases avoid touching clothing with your bare hands.

(e) Spillage on floor, work surfaces, etc.

(e) If the spillage is *major*, use absorbent material to soak up excess blood. This should be treated as CONTAMINATED MATERIAL and handled as in (d).

All areas where blood has been spilt, whether major or minor, should be thoroughly washed in a solution of hot water and bleach (1 part bleach to 10 parts water).

arrange disposal by your local Council. If the spillage is *minor*, wash in as high a temperature as the fabric will allow in a washing machine. In both cases avoid touching clothing with your bare hands.

(e) Spillage on floor, work surfaces, etc.

(e) If the spillage is *major*, use absorbent material to soak up excess blood. This should be treated as CONTAMINATED MATERIAL and handled as in (d).

All areas where blood has been spilt, whether major or minor, should be thoroughly washed in a solution of hot water and bleach (1 part bleach to 10 parts water).

Table 6.1 continued

Hepatitis B		HIV	
Method of transmission	Good hygienic practice	Method of transmission	Good hygienic practice
	NB. On special floor surfaces, clean as per manufacturers' guidelines. In all cases avoid touching contaminated areas with your bare hands.		NB. On special floor surfaces, clean as per manufacturers' guidelines. In all cases avoid touching contaminated areas with your bare hands.
(f) Toothbrushes and razors.	(f) People should be discouraged from sharing such items as toothbrushes and razors because of the risk from infected blood contamination.	(f) Toothbrushes and razors.	(f) People should be discouraged from sharing such items as toothbrushes and razors because of the risk from infected blood contamination.
2 Vomit (a) On clothing	(a) Contaminated clothing should be carefully removed. Excess vomit should be carefully removed and flushed down the toilet.	2 Vomit (a) On clothing	(a) Contaminated clothing should be carefully removed. Excess vomit should be carefully removed and flushed down the toilet.

Clothing can then be washed in a washing machine at the highest temperature possible for the fabric. Where possible, avoid touching contaminated material with your bare hands.

(b) On floors and work surfaces

Excess vomit should be carefully removed and flushed down the toilet, using absorbent material such as paper towels. Surfaces should then be thoroughly cleaned as per 1(e).

(a) It is important to ensure that all cutlery and crockery are thoroughly washed using hot soapy water.

(b) People should be discouraged from

3 Saliva

Clothing can then be washed in a washing machine at the highest temperature possible for the fabric. Where possible, avoid touching contaminated material with your bare hands.

(b) Excess vomit should be carefully removed and flushed down the toilet, using absorbent material such as paper towels. Surfaces should then be thoroughly cleaned as per 1(e).

(b) On floors and work surfaces

3 Saliva

(a) NOT APPLICABLE (Although there has been no evidence of transmission of HIV through saliva, good hygienic practice is advisable.)

Table 6.1 continued

Hepatitis B		HIV	
Method of transmission	*Good hygienic practice*	*Method of transmission*	*Good hygienic practice*
	sharing such items as toothbrushes and razors because of the risk from infected-saliva contamination.		(b) NOT APPLICABLE (Although there has been no evidence of transmission of HIV through saliva, good hygienic practice is advisable.)
4 Sexual activity and other methods of transmission not specifically mentioned in this handout	There are a variety of leaflets and materials available relating to safe sex practices and the transmission route between mother and unborn child.	4 Sexual activity and other methods of transmission not specifically mentioned in this handout	There are a variety of leaflets and materials available relating to safe sex practices and the transmission route between mother and unborn child.

Source: Patterson and Pattison, 1990.

APPENDIX 6.3 CASUALTY CARDS

Table 6.2 Casualty card: drug overdose in toilet

Condition	Signs and symptoms	Action
Drug overdose in toilet	Unconscious	Remove patient from toilet, place in recovery position
	Pulse possibly increased rate	
	Respiration possibly laboured	Remove restriction on arm
	Possible needle marks on arms	*Safety* Be careful of needle and other equipment possible danger from hepatitis and HIV
	Pupils pinpointed but will increase (dilate) after 8 hours from last fix	
	Note. Will not pinpoint if taken with stimulants (e.g. amphetamines, cocaine, etc.)	Always seek medical advice

Source: Patterson and Pattison, 1990.

Table 6.3 Casualty card: known drug user – cut on hand

Condition	Signs and symptoms	Action
Known drug user – cut on hand	Severe bleeding from wound	*Safety* Consider risk of infection from blood
	Will probably be co-operative but may be confused	Apply direct pressure to wound. Elevate and treat with wound dressing
	Might know if suffering from hepatitis and/or HIV	Take to health centre or hospital for further treatment

Source: Patterson and Pattison, 1990.

Table 6.4 Casualty card: tablets and alcohol, vomiting

Condition	Signs and symptoms	Action
Tablets and alcohol	Face flushed Pulse increased Speech slurred May become sick May go unconscious	Calm approach. Talk to *NOT* at him/her If sick – clear airway. If unconscious put in recovery position Can you cope in project or do you require assistance from relatives, friends, ambulance or police? May take several hours to return to normal
Vomiting	Casualty may have vomited and be unable to clear their airway. Signs of laboured breathing and appear pale Casualty may be trying to clear his/her airway by coughing May be in a sleep-like state or even unconscious	Clear vomit from face and neck. Check and clear mouth. Extend neck to open airway. If not breathing begin mouth-to-mouth resuscitation If breathing, place in recovery position and check condition until casualty recovers *Do not leave casualty until he/she is fully recovered* If you have to do mouth-to-mouth or are unsure of patient's condition seek medical aid

Source: Patterson and Pattison, 1990.

Table 6.5 Casualty card: amphetamine user

Condition	Signs and symptoms	Action
Amphetamine user	Increase in heart rate and breathing; appetite plus desire to drink and sleep suppressed	Calm approach
	Initial feelings of increased energy, confidence and physical and mental capacity	Try to reassure
	As body's energy stores become depleted, may become restless, anxious and agitated. (High doses, particularly when repeated regularly, can produce panic, hallucinations and 'psychosis'.)	Listen to what is being said – can you and user cope with what is going on, or do 'psychotic' symptoms necessitate medical intervention?
	Effects last about 3/4 hours	Are there friends or relatives who can cope more appropriately?
	On withdrawal from successive or long-term use may feel very hungry, exhausted and depressed	It is important to respond to requests for food, drink (non-alcoholic) and rest

Source: Patterson and Pattison, 1990.

Table 6.6 Casualty card: solvent user, cut to head

Condition	Signs and symptoms	Action
Solvent user (aerosol, e.g. hair spray) Cut to head	Disorientated. Behaviour similar to being drunk – euphoria, dizziness, may feel sick, etc. with related risks	If indoors, *open* windows for ventilation to protect you and the solvent user from continued effect of fumes
	Effects normally last from 15–45 minutes	Try to reassure and stay calm – do not raise your voice or initiate aggressive behaviour
	Breathing and heart rate slower Possible marks around mouth and nose – often tell-tale smell of solvents	Do not criticize hallucinations; they may be real enough to user; remember the effects will wear off soon
	May experience hallucinations – these may be pretence, enhanced by other users Bleeding from wound – user may not be aware of this	Try and control bleeding by direct pressure and apply wound dressing, if possible. Consider sending to hospital re. wound to head but wait until solvent effects wear off, if possible

Source: Patterson and Pattison, 1990.

Table 6.7 Casualty card: epilepsy (major)

Condition	Signs and symptoms	Action
Epilepsy (major)	May get warning (normally very brief) i.e. a noise, taste, sight or sensation	Create space, move all objects from area
		DO NOT restrict movements unless to prevent injury
	Will go rigid and fall to ground. Breathing may cease	Protect head
	Muscles relax and begin convulsive (jerky) movements. Breathing may sound noisy. Froth which may be bloodstained might appear from mouth	When fit finishes, place in recovery position, clear airway
		Check pockets for card. If present follow instructions
	Bladder and/or bowels may suffer loss of control	If only one fit occurs wait for person to recover
	Muscles cease movement and patient will normally sleep	Only send to hospital if it is not known if person suffers from epilepsy, or if he/she takes more than one fit or if he/she is injured
		REMAIN CALM

Source: Patteron and Pattison, 1990.

REFERENCES

Patterson, V. and Pattison, D. (1990) *Drug Awareness and First Aid Video Teaching Pack*, Edinburgh: Drugs Training Project and Scottish Branch of the British Red Cross, with SHEG.

Van Heiningen, R.M. (1989) Paper 'Drugs & HIV in the Netherlands' given in Blackpool at The Challenge of HIV Conference organised by the Drug Trainers Forum.

OTHER TEACHING MATERIALS

Institute for the Study of Drug Dependence Overdose Aid wallchart.

Marsden, N. (1978) *Diagnosis Before First Aid*, Edinburgh: Churchill Livingstone.

Ward Gardner, A. and Roylance, P.J. (1980) *New Essential First Aid*, London: Pan.

Chapter 7

Harm reduction (with Andy Fox, Bridge Project, Ayr)

WHAT IS HARM REDUCTION?

Harm reduction means essentially working with drug users on *their* terms. By enabling drug users to make realistic choices concerning their future drug use they are helped to minimise any damage to themselves, their families and friends, and the wider community where they can be recognised as a benefit rather than a cost. Working with harm reduction means that drug workers need to be clear about their role in such a client-centred approach. It is probable that most drug workers already employ harm-reduction strategies in their daily contact with drug users, although they may not formally recognise this. In fact, harm reduction as a viable method of working with drug users has been recognised since the Rolleston Committee of 1926 made it legal for doctors to prescribe opiates not only to treat but also to maintain drug 'addicts' – what has been called 'The British System'. It is only now, however, that harm reduction is 'emerging from the closet'. Ironically it is mainly the onset of HIV and AIDS that has currently given credibility and acceptance to this client-centred approach within treatment and rehabilitation. Even the government, by funding and legitimising needle-exchange schemes has given tacit approval to harm reduction as a principle for working with drug users. However, harm reduction should not only be related to reduced health risks, particularly in relation to HIV and AIDS, but *any* drug-related harm.

Before going on to look at what types of drug-related harm we should be trying to reduce, it is important to briefly relate this model of working with drug users to the traditional abstinence-oriented models of working with addictions.

The abstinence-oriented approach evolved out of a medical view of addiction as an illness. This approach can take choice, and therefore power, away from the client and imposes a view of drug-taking that may be meaningless for many users, e.g. the Minnesota Method and Narcotics Anonymous which are both derived from the basic principles of the AA movement. This model can, for example, set up both the worker and the client for failure in that it assumes the possibility that someone can just 'give up' their drug use. It does not allow for controlled or recreational drug use, or relapse, which in a harm-reduction model would be seen as possible stages in the process towards abstinence. Rather, they are seen as failures with concomitant guilt for both worker and client. The worker may then perceive themselves as working with a 'constantly relapsing client' which can be deskilling for the worker and will simply reinforce negative patterns for drug users.

Harm reduction can be seen as a goal in itself as well as a stage in the process of change towards abstinence. Because it is a person-centred method of working, it goes at the client's pace which is a recognised social work principle (Egan, 1981; Hollis, 1964). It is a method of working that takes account of the client's needs as its primary goal.

WHAT TYPE OF DRUG-RELATED HARM?

There are two fundamental forms of harm that can be associated with illicit drug use – individual harm and harm to the community. It may be that by reducing the harm to the individual there will be a resulting reduction in harm to the community. For example, a user who returns their needles and syringes to a needle exchange reduces the possible number of these items found discarded in public places. This, in turn, reduces the risk of children playing with such items.

Community harm

For example:

Discarded injection equipment in public places.
Violence between drug users and/or drug dealers.
Theft and robbery.
Prostitution: users prostituting themselves to obtain money for drugs.

Spread of HIV and other viruses through sexual contact.

Excessive costs of police, prisons, court systems, health and social services.

Cost of people being unable to creatively and productively participate in society.

Note that the sale of stolen property and prostitution only continue to be viable as sources of income because of a certain level of public demand for, acceptance of, and collusion with these illegal services (Box, 1983; Hobbs, 1988).

Individual harm

Individual harm can be separated into three main types – social and personal, legal, and health-related, although all three are inter-related.

1 *Social and personal harm.* Drug users are negatively stereotyped and stigmatised by society leading to feelings of low self-worth which in turn exacerbate relations between the drug user and the wider community. For example:

   Interpersonal relations with friends, family and employers may be harmed.

   Employment prospects can be damaged by having a criminal record related to drug use and by non-attendance at work due to intoxication.

   Educational prospects will be harmed if someone is using drugs chaotically. Access to further education may be restricted. Expulsion or absence from school or college also affects a young person's educational chances.

   Access to community resources may be restricted to known drug users, particularly youth provision. This can have a marked effect on the drug user's self-image and relationships with non-users, further reinforcing negative stereotypes.

2 *Legal harm.* Drug use as defined under the Misuse of Drugs Act 1971 is illegal. It is within these terms of reference that legal harm must be defined, and that can leave the drug user with a criminal record, imprisonment, fines and related social harm, e.g. difficulty in obtaining employment, housing, visas and a passport. Reducing legal harm can be difficult. It is important to discuss any planned harm-reduction strategies with the police and judiciary, e.g. diversion schemes; the police agreeing not to

harass needle exchange users or use injecting equipment as legal evidence; no legal action taken for possession of small amounts of cannabis for personal use.

3 *Health-related harm.* Health-related harm applies to physical and/or psychological harm. For example:

Overconsumption or accidentally overdosing can lead to physical damage and can possibly be fatal. High doses of drugs over long periods can seriously damage internal organs, e.g. link between long-term, heavy alcohol use and cirrhosis of the liver.

Operating machinery or driving a car while intoxicated is potentially dangerous not only to the user but to other people as well.

Young people experimenting with solvents often use their drugs in dangerous places like derelict buildings, or by a river or canal. Combined with intoxication, this can create a number of potentially harmful situations.

Ingestion often causes the most obvious and dramatic harm. As a method of ingestion, injection causes the most physical harm. Through unclean and infected equipment, blood poisoning and viruses can cause amputation and fatalities. Injection into inappropriate sites, i.e. groin, eyes, penis, vagina, hands, feet or jugular vein, is dangerous and can cause permanent damage. It is important that injectors learn to regularly change their injection site and inject less often if the site becomes infected. However, remember that other forms of ingestion, e.g. the smoking of *any* drug, can also be harmful.

Women are at further risk to their health, as regular use of opiates, barbiturates and other drugs will affect the menstrual cycle. Their periods may become unpredictable and erratic; they may stop for weeks, months, or even years, leading some women to a belief that they are infertile.

People using prostitution as a way of financing a drug habit increase the risk of sexually transmitted diseases, and for women this increases the chance of cervical cancer. Having a regular smear test should be recommended to any woman in this situation, as should protective types of contraceptives like condoms. (See *Changing Gear*, The Blenheim Project, 1988).

A low self-image through unemployment or poor personal relationships can be exacerbated by society once an individual has been labelled and stigmatised as a drug user. This can lead to increased stress levels which may cause an individual to change their drug taking from occasional or recreational use to a more chaotic pattern resulting in physiological, psychological or emotional harm.

The organic effects of psychoactive substances on the brain can, in a small percentage of heavy users, result in mental disturbances such as psychotic episodes, e.g. for very heavy users of amphetamines:

> toxic effects are liable to develop, including delusions, hallucinations and feelings of paranoia. Many experienced users are aware that their paranoia is drug induced, but sometimes these feelings lead to hostility as stimulant users defend themselves against imagined attacks. These symptoms will abate, but persist for a time after drugtaking has stopped. In a few people they develop into a psychotic state, from which it can take several months to recover.
>
> (ISDD, 1988: 8)

WHY HARM REDUCTION? IMPLICATIONS FOR POLICY AND PRACTICE

Policy

Attitudes to drug problems and responses to drug users and treatment change according to the prevailing political climate which is determined largely by politicians and multinational corporate interests and does not always reflect the community's best interests. What is needed is a coherent policy that incorporates harm reduction as a central strategy in working with drug users, whatever the prevailing political climate.

In Britain, for example, The Dangerous Drugs Acts of 1920 and 1923 emphasised penalising those who imported or produced certain drugs rather than the individuals who used them. The Misuse of Drugs Act of 1971, however, changed this emphasis by further criminalising the individual user, thus increasing related harm due to more stringent sentencing policy and court disposals. This Act has helped to fuel the common assumption that all use of illegal drugs is harmful and that all users of illegal drugs are problematic and should be stopped or locked up.

How does this fit in with the more liberal tradition of the 'British system', which emphasised treatment rather than punishment? On the one hand, drug policy in Britain has derived from this tradition, yet on the other it has followed the US by being firmly entrenched in a prohibitionist stance which criminalises drug users.

Note that current, prohibitionist drug laws and policies are likely to make drugs and their use *more*, rather than less, harmful. For example (a) the creation of a black market in drugs means an increase in prices, the likelihood that some users will turn to crime to maintain a costly habit, and that without any quality control 'street drugs' will be adulterated with substances that may be more harmful than the drugs themselves; (b) harsher sentencing and longer prison sentences for intravenous drug users increases the risk of HIV infection spreading in prisons with subsequent spread to the community outside prison through heterosexual transmission. They also help to create family- and community-related harm.

In Britain, then, there still remains confusion over the paradoxes and double standards of drug policy. For drug workers, the question is how far is your work practice determined by current policy? For example, is it a balance of care and control? Should you intervene in the case of recreational cannabis users? What should your role be when working with drug users?

Practice

As already stated harm reduction means accepting the drug user on their own terms and working with their needs and wants which may not be in keeping with government, social or project policy. For example, as a drug worker or project are you funded to stop people taking drugs or are you funded to work at the users' level helping them to reduce the harm involved in drug use? Are you there to meet the needs and wants of the individual user or the demands of the state to act as an agent of social control within a policy of criminalisation and eradication of drug use? Will practising harm reduction be seen by your managers and other agencies like the police as condoning and colluding with illegal drug use?

These are practical questions that drug workers need to answer for themselves. What is needed is a flexible and eclectic style of working that accepts that drug use is a complex, diverse form of human behaviour where no one method of intervention will solve the problem. Harm reduction is one such method of intervention which itself is flexible and eclectic and needs appropriate person-centred skills to be effective. The following points illustrate the benefits of harm reduction as a way of working with drug users:

1 The normality of drug use and experimentation among young people needs to be accepted by the worker. If they challenge this then they also challenge youth culture and therefore are at risk of losing their credibility with those youth groups who may be functioning outside the law. As Mark Gilman points out, one of the theories used to guide the practice of new drug services that emerged in the 1980s was that, 'the problem drug users of the 1980s are likely to be more numerous, more normal and younger than their 1960s and 1970s counterparts' (Gilman, 1989:9). Furthermore,

> though illicit drug use has not yet become typical amongst most British youths, it has become 'normalised' in the sense that the majority of 15–20-year-olds in urban areas such as London, Edinburgh and Merseyside are likely to have one or more friends who take drugs, and a substantial minority will be taking drugs such as cannabis and solvents on an experimental or recreational basis ... the present generation of drug using youths should not be abandoned to inappropriate primary prevention programmes, nor to the many preventable problems (e.g. overdose, infection, organic damage, accidents) that can occur because of a lack of knowledge about safe use procedures
>
> (Newcombe, 1987:10)

2 It has been suggested that 'addicts may mature out, or cease drug use as they get older, possibly because the social pressures that motivate addiction become less salient or more readily handled by the maturing addict' (Anglin et al., 1986).

Although this notion of 'the maturing out process' is not seen as adequate to describe the experiences of all long-term users who stop taking drugs (Waldorf, 1983), it is generally accepted as part of many drug careers. One of the main roles of the worker, then, is to ensure that as much information relating to drug use as possible is given to users who can then be supported in making rational choices not only about the drugs they use but the relative harm involved. This will go some way to ensure that when they reach the point in the maturing out process when they will seriously consider no longer using drugs as little irreversible damage as possible has been caused.

3 Harm reduction is easier for drug users to accept as it allows for gradual movement and change at *their* pace. As opposed to abstinence it does not expect people to make what may be perceived as a major leap in their drug use, their personal identity, and their everyday life style. This does not, however, mean that abstinence cannot be the final goal of any harm-reduction programme.

4 Harm reduction can promote a viable working relationship between the worker and the drug user who sees himself as having an equal amount of control over mutually agreed goals. To establish this relationship the user has to be asked about what *they* want to do and what *their* choice is about their future drug use. In reality it is likely that there will be a lot of testing out by both client and worker over what is meant by 'an equal amount of control'. This testing-out period may take a long time during which the worker's power and authority is likely to be questioned and challenged. During this period the client may leave the relationship several times before seeing the benefits. From this basis drug users can see themselves as being accepted on their own terms with their needs and wants being taken seriously. This, of course, necessitates a non-judgmental stance on the part of the worker and an acceptance on the part of the drug user that they have power and can make realistic decisions and choices. It is also a position that may take some time to arrive at, not just from the perspective of the worker, but also that of the drug user as it may challenge some drug users' perceptions of themselves as 'victims' or 'sick people' who neither have, nor want, any control over, or responsibility for, their lives.

> The role of the helper is not to choose which type of help is most suitable. It is to stand alongside the client as the stages of change are experienced, make information available to the client, help the decision-making process, and support the client's experiments in achieving change. The client is in the driving seat, not a passenger in the helper's car(e). The goals are chosen by the client, not imposed by the helper.
>
> (Shephard, 1990)

5 Harm reduction can empower generic workers, for example,

social workers, youth and community workers and health-care workers, to work effectively with drug users without the need to refer on to a specialist in the drug field. This presumes that generic workers, as well as specialist drug workers, are skilled in a range of person-centred treatment methods. By accepting harm reduction as a method of working, rather than abstinence, workers can have more realistic expectations of both the drug users they are working with *and* themselves. Working with mutually acceptable, achievable goals and minimising any sense of failure – even if these goals do not work – also means that workers reduce the risk of stress to themselves. Harm reduction is not just about reducing harm for drug users, it can also reduce stress-related harm for workers.

A HARM-REDUCTION COURSE MODEL

The following is a model for running a 2-day non-residential course on harm reduction for a group of 12–18 drug workers. A group of less experienced or knowledgeable workers will need at least one extra day of basic drug-awareness training *before* they come on this course. You need, therefore, to be able to assess workers' levels of experience and knowledge well before they come on the course.

Aim of the course

The general aim of the course is to enable workers to recognise and understand the issues and problems that may arise for them when working with a harm-reduction approach. Not all drug users when presenting for help will either want to stop using or will realistically be able to stop using. It is important that workers are able to recognise the harm that is associated with that use and are able to work towards a treatment aim that will reduce the harm to the individual, the family and the community.

The specific aims of the course are:

1 To extend participants' knowledge and understanding of drugs, drug users and associated harm,
2 To examine participants' attitudes to drugs and drug users,
3 To enable participants to assess the needs of drug users in relation to the type(s) of harm associated with their particular style of drug use,

Table 7.1 Programme for a 2-day harm-reduction course

Day 1	Day 2	
	Option 1	Option 2
Session 1 (a) Introduction and expectations (b) A historical perspective	Session 1 Short- and long-term goal setting (role play)	Session 1 Social and personal harm (role play)
COFFEE	COFFEE	COFFEE
Session 2 (a) Drugs, effects and related harm (b) What harm are we trying to reduce?	Session 2 Breakdown of resolution (role play)	Session 2 Legal harm (role play)
LUNCH	LUNCH	LUNCH
Session 3 Models of dependency	Session 3 Working with families and the community (role play)	Session 3 Health-related harm (role play)
TEA	TEA	TEA
Session 4 Assessing levels of use and the needs of the user – preparation for practical work in Day 2	Session 4 (a) Working with managers (b) Course feedback	Session 4 (a) Working with managers (b) Course feedback

4 To enable participants to develop a method of treatment aimed at achieving a less harmful form of drug use that will not compromise or collude with drug use,

5 To help managers support a harm reduction strategy as a viable aim for working with drug users.

Table 7.1 is the programme for the 2-day harm-reduction course. Note that there are two options for the second day and that the programme does not include a timetable. *You* should make decisions about the time needed for each session based on your level of knowledge and competence and your assessment of participants' needs. Each session is numbered, named and explained in the text.

A 2-DAY HARM-REDUCTION COURSE
THE REDUCTION AND MINIMISATION OF
DRUG-RELATED HARM

Day 1

Session 1

Introduction and expectations

See Chapter 4, p. 65 for an introduction exercise. It is useful to find out participants' expectations of the course. This should be based on their work with drug users and what they feel they need to know and want to learn from the course. One way of eliciting this information is to send out a short questionnaire 2–4 weeks before the course. Another is to spend about 15 minutes of this session carrying out a brainstorm exercise.

Whatever method is used you should spend some time talking to participants about whether or not their expectations will be met and guide people to resources that will meet their unmet expectations.

A historical perspective

This should be a short presentation which includes a question-and-answer session. It should focus on how and why current drugs legislation has evolved and how that legislation has shaped public and political attitudes towards drug users and their treatment,

particularly harm-reduction strategies.
Some historical areas you might want to focus on are:

The Opium trade in Britain in the 1800s
The Opium Wars
The Defence of the Realm Act 1916
The Rolleston Committee 1926
The Brain Committees 1958 and 1965
The Dangerous Drugs Acts 1920, 1923, 1951, 1964 and 1967
The Misuse of Drugs Act 1971
ACMD reports of the 1980s

If you have time, it is also useful to compare how legislation in
Britain has developed with legislation in the US or Holland, and to
what extent this has led to different perceptions of drug users and
treatment programmes in these countries.

[Holland] is the only country where the government itself
calmly supports peaceful approaches to drug problems and
openly opposes the very idea of war on drugs. The Dutch seem
to have dealt largely with the marijuana issue but have still not
solved all their difficulties with drugs. Yet their spirit of moder-
ation and experimentation is unmatched.

(Trebach, 1987: 376)

Some references you can use for this session include Berridge and
Edwards, 1987; Gossop, 1987; Stimson and Oppenheimer, 1982;
Trebach, 1982.

Session 2

If participants have not already completed a basic drug-awareness
day then you can use some of the exercises given in Chapter 3 for
this session or do a short input giving more detailed information
about possible harm. This can be taken from ISDD's *Drug Abuse
Briefing* and their Drug Misuse wallchart. This session should
enable people to think about what 'harm' means for them and how
they deal with it.

First, give a brief input on definitions and types of harm based
on 'What type of drug-related harm?' on pp. 125-8, this chapter.
Next, divide participants into two groups asking one group to
brainstorm and discuss question X and the other group to brainstorm and discuss question Y. Allow 30 minutes for this.

Question X. What behaviour of my client is acceptable to me and what is unacceptable?
Check whether this behaviour is normally unacceptable or only pertains to drug users.
Question Y. How do I keep my opinions to myself and not judge how a drug user is behaving?
Check how people cope with their feelings when they are confronted with behaviour that may be unacceptable to them. Allow time for feedback and discussion in the large group.

Session 3 Models of dependency

The main aim of this session is to provide participants with a practical model of drug use that will enable them to work with harm reduction as a method of treatment. If you think it is necessary, you can start the session by carrying out the dependency exercise on p. 27 of Chapter 2. This will raise several questions and issues that could be discussed, for example, what is the difference between dependence and addiction? Is dependence an inevitable consequence of long-term drug use? How do you distinguish between physical and psychological dependence? You can

	Benefits (Positives)	**Costs** (Negatives)
Short term	e.g. 'I like the effect' 'Drugs make me feel better' 'All my friends use'	e.g. Risk of infection through injecting Risk of accident or overdose Risk of arrest, prosecution and conviction
Long term	e.g. 'It's my career, identity' 'I've got my life together, I can cope'	e.g. Relationship difficulties Physical dependency

Note: Harm reduction is about aiming to eliminate the negatives of this pay-off chart.

Figure 7.1 Drug-use pay-off chart

then give a brief input outlining and comparing some of the more common models of dependency, for example, the medical model, the moral model and psychosocial models (Krivanek, 1988: 29–56). Suggest that what is needed is a model that does not judge or stigmatise the drug user but sees dependency as a form of human behaviour which, like many others, has costs and benefits. In the case of drug dependency the costs can be very high indeed, so reducing, or ideally eliminating, these costs should be the aim of treatment.

By using the pay-off chart in Figure 7.1 the worker can help their client to identify what it is they wish to change about their drug-using behaviour.

Session 4 Assessing levels of drug use and the needs of the user

This session, along with the pay-off chart in session 3, should be used to prepare participants for the more practical work they will be doing in Day 2. There are two sets of ideas you should introduce during this session:

1 Motivational interviewing
2 The process of change

Even if participants are familiar with these ideas it is useful to go over them again before the exercises are attempted.

Motivational interviewing

Motivational interviewing was first described as an integral part of a treatment approach by Miller in the following way:

> an approach based on principles of experimental social psychology, applying processes such as attribution, cognitive dissonance and self-efficacy. Motivation is conceptualised not as a personality trait, but as an interpersonal process. The model de-emphasises labelling and places heavy emphasis on individual responsibility and internal attribution change. Cognitive dissonance is created by contrasting ... the problem behaviour with ... awareness of the behaviour's negative consequences, and ... [channelled] towards a behaviour change solution, avoiding the 'short circuits' of low self-esteem, low self-efficacy and denial.
>
> (Miller, 1983)

Table 7.2 The characteristics of motivational interviewing

Motivational interviewing	Traditional approach
Individual responsibility	
Emphasis on personal choice regarding future use of heroin.	Emphasis on the disease of addiction which reduces personal choice.
Goal of treatment is negotiated based on data and preferences.	The treatment goal is always total and life-long abstinence.
Controlled heroin use is a possible goal though not optimal for all.	Controlled heroin use is dismissed as impossible.
Internal attribution	
The individual is seen as able to control and choose.	The individual is seen as helpless towards heroin and unable to control his/her own heroin use.
The interviewer focuses on eliciting the client's own statement of concern regarding the heroin use.	The interviewer presents perceived evidence to convince the client of his or her problem.
Denial/telling lies	
Denial and telling lies are seen as an interpersonal behaviour pattern (communication) influenced by the interviewer's behaviour.	Denial and telling lies are seen as a personal trait of the heroin addict/junkie, requiring heavy confrontation by the interviewer.
Lies and denial are met with reflections.	Lies and denial are met with argument/correction.
Labelling	
There is a general de-emphasis on labels. Confessions of being a junkie or being an irresponsible heroin addict are seen as irrelevant.	There is a heavy emphasis on acceptance of the person as a junkie or an addict.
Objective data of impairment are presented in a low-key fashion, not imposing any conclusion on the client.	Objective data of impairment are presented in a confrontational fashion; as proof of a progressive disease and the necessity of complete abstinence.

Source: van Bilsen and van Emst, 1989: 36.

The chart on Table 7.2 contrasts some of the key principles of motivational interviewing with the more traditional approach to working with drug users. Note how these principles will affect the relationship between the worker and the drug user.

You can use the chart in Table 7.2 to carry out the following exercise.

Exercise   Each participant should carry out an analysis of the costs and benefits for themselves as workers of both the motivational method of interviewing *and* the traditional approach. Allow 10–15 minutes for this exercise and ask participants to keep their notes.

As an optional extra you could now divide the participants into two groups and do the following exercise.

Exercise   Group 1 should make out a case for using motivational interviewing and group 2 should make out a case for using the traditional approach. Allow 20 minutes.
The two groups should then be given 5 minutes each to present their case. Following questions and answers of each group plus a general discussion, a vote could be taken to establish what method of interviewing is preferred. Having a vote is an optional ending.

The process of change

In assessing a drug user's motivation to change it is useful to use the model in Figure 7.2, adapted from the work of Prochaska and DiClemente.

1 **Precontemplation** is the stage where drug users do not perceive they have a problem with their drug use although others around them may be disapproving. They may well have been coerced by others to seek help because even at this stage there may be some harm related to social stability and relationship with family or friends.

2 **Contemplation** is the stage where the drug user begins to look at the costs and benefits of their drug use. There may well be evidence of poor health, financial problems, interpersonal

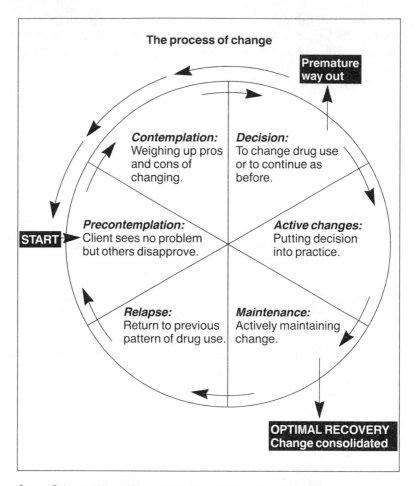

Source: Bolton and Watt, 1989:8, adapted from the work of Prochaska and DiClemente.

Figure 7.2 The process of change model.

difficulties etc., but the drug user still identifies positive aspects of their drug use that helps them to cope with everyday stress and strain.

3 **Decision** is the stage at which the drug user has decided what they want to do in terms of realistic change. It is likely that drug users will not stay in this stage for long choosing either to return to precontemplation and previous levels of drug use *or* to move to the next stage of active change.

4 **Active change** is the stage at which the drug user takes action to put their decision into practice. Here the worker should be enabling the drug user to negotiate goals, for example, to stop injecting, to use a needle-exchange scheme, not to supplement a maintenance or reduction prescription.

5 **Maintenance.** The worker should now be introducing coping strategies to maintain the resolution to change. Relapse prevention techniques have been well documented by Marlatt and Gordon, 1985.

6 **Relapse** is the return to the drug use patterns of the prechange period. It is often unusual for a drug user to maintain the resolution to change. If a relapse does happen it should be treated as a learning experience and not a failure on behalf of the drug user *or* worker. Note that the occasional drug use episode does not amount to a relapse and should be learned from and dealt with in maintenance.

(Adapted from Bolton and Watt, 1989)

Using the pay-off chart to help the drug user identify the areas of their drug use they want to change, the worker can then explain each stage of the process-of-change model to the drug user in an effort to establish at what point they believe themself to be in their drug use.

Drug workers may make wrong assumptions about where their client is within this process. Many drug users will be either pre-contemplators or contemplators and may not yet be determined to change.

Drug users themselves may not be clear about what aspects of their drug use they are not happy with so the primary aim should be to help the drug user, by means of a costs-and-benefits exercise, to identify what they wish to change. It is then the role of the worker to help them achieve these changes. Note that stopping drug use may not enter into this negotiation at all.

To illustrate the above process for themselves participants can do the following exercise.

Cost-benefit exercise   Participants should be in pairs for this exercise. Each participant should be asked to choose something on which they are dependent and – using the pay-off chart (see Figure 7.1) to write down the costs and benefits of that dependency. With their partner they should then attempt to identify how they can reduce or eliminate the costs, whilst highlighting the benefits; what might prevent them achieving change; and how they would cope with a breakdown in their resolution. The time allowed for this exercise is 30 minutes. Time should then be allowed for a general discussion in the main group.

Day 2

There are four sessions in Day 2, with two available options. Option 1 is best used with experienced drug workers; option 2 with multidisciplinary groups and non-specialist generic workers.

Option 1

For the first three sessions you should work with one case study. You can ask participants to bring to the course a case of their own that they feel is unresolved, although it is also useful to have some other case studies available.

Session 1   Short- and long-term goal-setting

The aim of this first session is by using role-play exercises to move a drug-using client along through the process of change by helping them identify what it is they wish to change. Some of these changes will be small and immediate, e.g. 'I want to learn how to filter my drugs', and some changes will take more time, e.g. 'I want to stop injecting opiates and to use less speed.' These two changes will require different approaches.

Role-play exercise   Divide the participants into groups of three and give each group a case study to role play. Allow time for people to brief themselves on the case before getting into role. Each person in a group will play one of the following roles:

1 The client

2 The counsellor
3 The observer

The 'client' will present his or her case. It is the role of the 'coun-sellor' to help them identify the costs and benefits of their presented drug use and from that negotiate what changes they can make both in the short term and the long term. Long-term goals will only be achieved through setting short-term goals so emphasis should be placed on the short term.

The counsellor will help the client to identify not only what they want to change but also how they see that change occurring and what is likely to get in the way of change. The counsellor has access to a prescribing GP and should use this if necessary.

The 'observer' should be quietly making notes on how they see the relationship developing. Allow up to 30 minutes for the role play itself.

Debriefing

Next bring all the groups of three back together and allow each group some time to feed back. The client should say how they felt the session had gone, whether or not the most appropriate changes had been identified, and whether they would be able to achieve the short-term goals.

The counsellor should say how they felt during the interview, did they feel at ease, did they feel they were supporting and helping, or directing and controlling? Check with the observer, what did they see happening, what would they have done differently if they had been the counsellor? Do this for each group, taking notes for yourself, then allow time for general discussion.

Session 2 Breakdown of resolution

People should keep the roles they had in Session 1. The client will need to be primed to *not* achieve one or two of the changes agreed in Session 1 and to consider why.

Using the same role-play characters, the client should present the problems and the counsellor will need to help the person identify what cues moved them to return to former drug-taking patterns, e.g. a return to injecting; a return to sharing injecting equipment; getting an abscess through unclean injecting equipment.

Their task is to help the client identify what else they need to maintain the changes they wish to make. This means that renegotiation of goals may have to take place as they may not have been realistic in the first place. Allow up to 30 minutes for the role play. Now carry out the same debriefing as before.

Session 3 Working with families and the community

The role of the observer should now change. They will become a family member, e.g. partner, parent, or sibling. The client will need to brief the family member about their role in this session.

The aim is for the counsellor to want to encourage the family member to help the client maintain the changes. The counsellor will have to help the family member to understand the changes the client wants to make. The counsellor should also enable the client to talk more freely to the family member about their drug use and their long-term goals. Allow up to 30 minutes for the role play.

Debriefing

The debriefing will be slightly different this time. Start with the family member and check out how they felt about what was happening – did they feel they had a better understanding of the issues, of the client's drug use and the short- and long-term goals? Then check out how the client felt about what was happening – did they feel that they were supported by the counsellor and the family member? Did the counsellor feel they had achieved their goal; what was difficult about the session; what would they have done differently?

Allow some time for an open discussion, bringing together the main points of all three sessions. Check out whether the participants achieved what they needed, e.g. do they feel they were able to use the material from the previous day to affect the changes?

Note. There are other ways of organising the preceding role plays. For example, when working with a multidisciplinary group or generic workers, you can divide participants into larger groups. It may be useful to have a trainer in the role of facilitator/observer to supplement the group's knowledge. The other members of the group can be observers and/or other family members in role play. Remember this will necessitate more time and the size of these larger groups will be determined by the number of trainers working on the course.

Session 4   Working with managers

It is important to be clear about the difficulties of changing the attitudes of managers and colleagues if this needs to happen. If the operational policy is different to that of a harm-reduction strategy then negotiation will have to take place. At this stage you should engage the group in a brief discussion to determine their past, present or expected difficulties in implementing harm-reduction strategies. Now do the following exercise.

Exercise   Divide participants into groups of four or five. Each group should elect a facilitator/recorder who will take notes and feedback to the main group. Make sure flipcharts and felt-tip pens are available.

The task is for each group to discuss the following questions:

To implement a harm-reduction strategy there will need to be changes in our working method. What changes will be achievable with minimum fuss? What do we need to happen to enable our managers to understand the process and what will hinder this?

Allow 30 minutes for this, then each group should have 10 minutes to feedback. Your role is to encourage open discussion within each group and to encourage people to help one another to come to some consensus about how they will approach their colleagues and managers.

Option 2

There are four sessions in this option, Session 4 being identical to Session 4 in Option 1.

Session 1   Social and personal harm

Drawing on the material from Day 1, you should put together a case study that is predominantly concerned with social and personal harm. Use a similar role-play format to Option 1, that is, groups of three with members playing client, counsellor, and observer roles. The aim of the counsellor is to help identify the social and personal harm, why that harm has arisen and how best they can tackle the issues. What will get in the way of achieving

change and how should they proceed? Give each group the same
case study and allow up to 30 minutes for the role play.

Debriefing

Only one group should report back. You should then encourage
open discussion and draw out the main points from the members
of the other small groups. Check whether the other groups
approached the problem in the same way and whether they came
to different conclusions.

Session 2 Legal harm

Drawing on the material from the section on legal harm put
together another case study highlighting the legal harm associated
with drug use. For example, you could consider the possible effects
of a criminal record – loss of employment, access to passports and
visas, credit facilities and a driving licence. With the same groups
and the same format as Session 1, the counsellor should help to
clarify the effects of the legal harm, how this has affected
relationships with other people, and what the client would want to
change.

The aim is for the counsellor to help the client, first, to avoid
more legal harm and, second, to change how they feel about what
has happened to them. Allow up to 30 minutes for the role play.

Debriefing

Same format as Session 1, but this time another group should give
feedback.

Session 3 Health-related harm

Using the material from the section on health-related harm, choose
either physical or psychological damage and build up a case study
that will draw out the harm. Do not make the case study too
complex. It is important to be clear about what drugs are being
used, how long they have been used and how they are being
ingested, e.g. a heroin user who has been injecting regularly for 5
years presenting with abscesses or septicaemia; a user who has
been snorting amphetamines on a recreational basis for 2 years and

is beginning to suffer from mild panic attacks when coming down from the drug.

Again, the format is the same as Sessions 1 and 2. This time the aim of the counsellor is to identify the harm and then help the client to look at ways they can reduce the damage. Any existing damage must be dealt with, so referral to other agencies is paramount (or other team members, e.g. a doctor, a community psychiatric nurse). Allow up to 30 minutes for this role play.

Debriefing

The feedback process is the same as for previous sessions. Again, choose a different group from Sessions 1 and 2.

Session 4 Working with managers

This session should be the same as Session 4 in Option 1.

A FOLLOW-UP TO THIS COURSE (see timetable in Table 7.3)

As with other skills-based training courses, there needs to be a follow-up in order to consolidate learning and to look at any problems that may have arisen. Here is one possible outline for a one-day follow-up that has the following aims:

1 To identify what skills have been employed in working with drug users to minimise drug-related harm.
2 To identify and clarify any problems and difficulties that have arisen and go some way to resolving them.
3 To identify what helped people in using harm-reduction techniques and strategies.
4 To investigate what other resources could be used in order to continue in a more effective manner.

Given these aims the day should of course remain flexible in order to take in the needs of the participants.

As harm reduction becomes more acceptable you should help and encourage people to understand and work with the whole scope of harm reduction, that is, individual *and* community harm, social *and* personal harm, legal harm *and* health-related harm. This means you could think about creating training events around the

Table 7.3 Harm-reduction course: a 1-day follow-up

Session 1 Introduction
           Expectations of participants
           Summary of main points from previous course

Tea/coffee
Session 2 Investigate practice implications (small groups)
           Question 1 What did we find useful in implementing harm
                       reduction?
           Question 2 What has prevented us from implementing harm
                       reduction effectively?

Lunch
Session 3 Developing local educational material (small groups)
           Question 1 How have we attempted to do this?
           Question 2 What resources will we need to do this
                       effectively?

Tea/coffee
Session 4 Open discussion – where do we go from here?
             (For example, identifying future needs in relation to
             management practice and training)

following topics, for example: Drugs, Drug Users and the Law;
The Community's Response to Drug Use; Employment and
Education for Drug Users; Interpersonal Skills for Drug Users;
Safer Drug Use – including injection techniques; Working with
Women's Drug Use.

As already stated, what is needed at all levels, national, regional
and local, is a coherent drug policy that incorporates harm
reduction as a central strategy in working with drug users, whatever the prevailing political climate. Drug workers, and volunteers,
will need support, encouragement and back-up resources from
managers to work their way through the paradoxes and in-
consistencies inherent in the practice of harm reduction within
most current drug policies. However, it is the benefits of harm
reduction as a realistic way of working with drug users that needs
to be kept uppermost in mind. A harm-reduction approach:

1 Accepts drug users on their own terms and works with their
   needs and wants. It allows for gradual movement and realistic
   change at *their* pace.
2 Accepts the normality of drug use and experimentation among

many young people. Workers can maintain credibility with those youth groups functioning outside the law.

3 Accepts that many drug users will naturally 'mature-out' of a drug-taking career.

4 Can promote a viable working relationship between the worker and the drug user.

5 Can empower generic workers to work effectively with drug users without the need to refer on to a specialist in the drug field.

REFERENCES

Anglin, M., Brecht, M.L. and Woodward, J.A. (1986) 'An empirical study of maturing out – conditional factors', *The International Journal of the Addictions* 21 (2).

Berridge, V. and Edwards, G. (1987) *Opium and the People: Opiate Use in Nineteenth Century England,* New Haven: Yale University Press.

Blenheim Project (1988) *Changing Gear,* London: Blenheim Project.

Bolton, K. and Watt, R. (1989) 'Motivating change', *Druglink: The Journal on Drug Misuse in Britain,* 4 (4).

Box, S. (1983) *Power, Crime and Mystification,* London: Tavistock.

Egan, G. (1981) *The Skilled Helper: A Model for Systematic Helping and Interpersonal Relating,* Monterey, CA: Brooks/Cole.

Gilman, M. (1989) 'The mystery of the single appointment!', *Mersey Drugs Journal* 2: 9.

Gossop, M. (1987) *Living with Drugs,* London: Wildwood House, second edition.

Hobbs, D. (1988) *Doing the Business,* Oxford: Clarendon Press.

Hollis, F. (1964) *Casework: A Psychosocial Therapy,* New York: Random House.

Institute for the Study of Drug Dependence (1988) *Drug Abuse Briefing,* London: ISDD.

Institute for the Study of Drug Dependence (1989) Drug Misuse wallchart, London: ISDD.

Krivanek, J. (1988) *Addictions,* Sydney: Allen & Unwin.

Marlatt, G. and Gordon, J. (1985) *Relapse Prevention,* London: Guildford.

Miller, W.R. (1983) 'Motivational interviewing with problem drinkers', *Behavioural Psychotherapy* 11: 147–72.

Newcombe, R. (1987) 'High time for harm reduction', *Druglink* 2 (1), Jan/Feb.

Prochaska, J. and DiClemente, C. (1981) 'Measuring the process of change', paper presented at the annual meeting of the International Council of Psychologists, Los Angeles.

Shephard, A. (1990) *Substance Dependency: A Professional Guide,* Birmingham: Venture Press.

Stimson, G.V. and Oppenheimer, E. (1982) *Heroin Addiction: Treatment and Control in Britain*, London: Tavistock.

Trebach, A. (1982) *The Heroin Solution*, New Haven: Yale University Press.

Trebach, A. (1987) *The Great Drug War*, New York: Macmillan.

van Bilsen, H. and van Emst, A. (1989) 'Motivating heroin users for change' in G. Bennett (ed.) *Treating Drug Abusers*, London: Routledge.

Waldorf, D. (1983) 'Natural recovery from opiate addiction: some social-psychological processes of untreated recovery', *Journal of Drug Issues*, Spring.

Chapter 8

Training the trainers

With the increasing number of trainers being employed in the drug field and the high expectations of both local authority and voluntary sector employers that practitioners can also provide training, drug training has expanded considerably over the last ten years. The increased awareness within society generally about drug problems has also produced a demand from community groups for drug training, to help them understand the causes and attempt to prevent any increase in local problems. There has been a similar demand from workers outside the drug field.

Whether they have any training experience or not, many drug workers find themselves having to offer training of some type to community groups and other workers. Similarly trainers and educators outside the drug field are having to consider how best to offer drug training to those for whom they are responsible, e.g. trainers and educators in social work, community education, health services, the AIDS field, prisons and the teaching professions.

As the need for drug training has increased, the number of training packs has expanded, but those expected to use these packs may find difficulty in deciding which of them is most appropriate to their needs. (See Chapter 2, Appendix 2.1 for a list of drug training packs.) Drug workers may have received drug awareness and other basic training, although this is not always the case. Although they may have the practical skills in working with drug users they will not necessarily have the training skills to translate their knowledge of drugs into a positive learning experience for other people. Trainers in other disciplines as well as lecturers in higher education offering professional qualifying courses may have the training and teaching skills, but they will not necessarily have the drug knowledge nor the information as to what constitutes appropriate drug training. Drugs, like topics such as racism, sexism, and AIDS, can therefore become marginalised because teachers or trainers may feel inexperienced, deskilled and lacking in confidence to teach about this subject (See Chapter 3, pp. 34–5 re. the similar effect on generic workers).

Although there is no real agreement, those employed as drug trainers would probably agree that the basic philosophy behind good drug training is:

→ The exploration of people's *attitudes* towards drugs and drug users.
→ *Knowledge* and *information* enhancement.
→ *Skills* development.*

In Scotland, for example, there has been an attempt by drug trainers to follow as far as possible this philosophy. This was developed through discussion with other drug trainers and the Scottish Health Education Group, and followed the approach taken in drug education in Holland since the 1970s (De Haes and Schuurman, 1975; De Haes, 1986).

This approach has been passed on to drug workers and other professionals through 'training the trainers' courses which attempt to offer a framework for considering not only how to do drug training, but also what the philosophy behind it should be. The two groups of people who benefit most from such courses are:

1 Drug workers who have a responsibility for training.
2 Trainers who have a responsibility for other workers in contact with drug users.

However, different people may have different needs from this course (see, for example, Figure 8.1).

The course layouts which follow take account of the differing needs of participants, so, although both are entitled 'Training the Trainers', the content is not the same. Both were designed following negotiations with either the participants – in the case of the Course for Drug Workers – or the Sponsor – in the case of the Course for Trainers (see Chapter 1, p. 4).

The Course for Drug Workers was designed following requests from workers who were finding that their managers expected them not only to work with drug users, but also to train community groups and professionals in their locality. Participants' needs were

Drug workers

Have the drug knowledge and the practice skills of working with drug users

Needs
(a) Training and teaching skills
(b) An opportunity to practise these skills
(c) Knowledge of what training and teaching packs and exercises are effective/appropriate
(d) Knowledge of other appropriate resources
(e) An opportunity to learn about course design
(f) An opportunity to examine the aims, objectives and goals of drug training

Other trainers

Have the training and teaching skills

Needs
(a) Drug knowledge
(b) An opportunity to test out that knowledge
(c) Knowledge of what training and teaching packs and exercises are effective/appropriate
(d) Knowledge of other appropriate resources
(e) Ways of accumulating further information
(f) An opportunity to examine the aims, objectives and goals of drug training

Figure 8.1   The needs of drug workers and other trainers

*See the Advisory Council on the Misuse of Drugs Report, *Problem Drug Use: A Review of Training* (1990), London: HMSO. The report was published after this handbook was written.

ascertained through a pre-course questionnaire and conversations with those who were to attend the course. The follow-up was designed based on the feedback received at the end of Part 1. All participants attended on a voluntary basis and there were no obvious hidden agendas, other than participants' frustration at being expected to undertake so much training as part of their work. This was particularly true amongst those working in the statutory sector.

The Course for Trainers was designed following a request from a national sponsoring body. Negotiation was with this organisation and the regional managers of those who were to be participants. A clear remit was given to the trainers by the sponsor but unfortunately that same remit was not necessarily given to all the participants by the sponsor – this was established early on in the course and had to be resolved before any course work could be attempted. Had this not been done, the hidden agendas of the participants plus their fantasies of what the hidden agendas were of the sponsor would have interfered with the course. Some participants attended on a voluntary basis and some on an involuntary basis. This was following assurances from the sponsor that all participants came voluntarily. Again this was discussed with the participants in an attempt to clarify the position for everyone, and was included in the final report to the sponsor along with the concerns about the unclear remit. Amendments to the course design were made as the course progressed to take account of participants' needs. These had been supposedly identified beforehand by the sponsor, but it is unwise to presume that a sponsor necessarily knows the training needs of those sent on courses.

These kinds of problems are not unusual on courses where negotiation is done with the sponsor rather than the participants. It is important to be aware of hidden agendas and to take account of those who do not want to be there. These participants may not be motivated and may be resistant to learning. Their emotions, particularly anger, may create a barrier on the course which must be dealt with, through discussion, before the work can continue. If their feelings are acknowledged, it may help them to be more receptive to the learning process.

On any 'Training the Trainers' course, participants need more than just the knowledge of what are good exercises to use. It is essential that they have the experience of being trainers, and of using such exercises. They need to practise how to use exercises in small groups and where necessary how to give presentations on such subjects as 'drugs and their effects'. 'Training the Trainers' courses should offer a supportive environment where it is safe to take risks and make mistakes. Trainers can facilitate this by talking with participants about mistakes they have made on courses, by sharing their own anxieties and discussing difficulties they have encountered and problems they have had to resolve. Remember that trainers are role models on courses, and it is important to share this with the prospective trainers. People bring their childhood experiences of learning particularly of schools and teachers to adult education, and this can sometimes be a barrier to their receptiveness to new ideas. Participants on 'Training the Trainers' courses need to be aware of how they present themselves as trainers; whether they simply recreate the negative experiences of childhood learning, or whether they offer an opportunity for people to learn as adults where support and understanding should be the norm.

Learning involves change and new trainers need to be encouraged to recognise that in themselves and in those they teach. Change can sometimes be painful, so support is essential. People also need time to identify what they have learned and to discuss this with others. If this is included in the 'Training the Trainers' course, then hopefully participants will learn that this is essential on courses they will in turn design. For example, on Day 2 of Part 1 of the course for drug workers, 3 hours is given for presentation, discussion and debriefing (Sessions 6 and 7) following the exercise on 'Organising, Designing and Presenting a Course'. This not only allows time to consider what has been learnt, but also to look at the differing needs of the various groups for whom the courses are designed.

Before considering the two 'Training the Trainers' courses in detail, it is worth mentioning some aspects of course presentation which may be forgotten, but which are important to include. The aims of any course should be made clear both in the written information sent out in advance, and again during the 'Introductions' session. This gives both trainers and participants a means of gauging, both during and at the end of the course, whether these have been achieved. Everyone should also be made aware of the explicit and implicit ground rules and course procedures during the introductory session. Most course rules are implicit, but some may need to be clearly stated, for example:

1 No drink or drugs allowed on premises.
2 We would encourage and expect participants to be able to engage in course work at all times – and not to be incapacitated through alcohol or any other drugs, e.g. hangover next morning or excessive lunchtime drinking.
3 Either (a) everything discussed on this course is to be treated confidentially or (b) everything discussed on this course is open unless expressly requested to be kept confidential.

Although these 'Training the Trainers' courses are designed to look primarily at 1-day courses on drugs and their effects, it will be important to discuss what to do on other shorter training inputs participants may be asked to undertake. For example, how would they put an afternoon workshop together, or even a 1-hour session? Ensure that course participants also understand the language of training, e.g. what do words such as workshop, plenary and didactic mean?

START AS YOU MEAN TO CONTINUE

Beginnings and endings of courses are important, but are often overlooked in the trainer's haste to reach the substantive content. The beginning of a training event sets the scene for the rest of the course, so the introductions and first impressions are all too important.

EACH ENDING (OF A COURSE) IS A NEW BEGINNING (FOR THOSE ON IT)

At the end of a course, participants need time to reflect on what they have learned. They need to think of not only what they are taking back with them, but also what they are going back to. This is particularly necessary at the end of a residential course where a participant may have experienced personal growth through learning. They need to consider how they will share this with family and co-workers, and what the effect of this might be. Time should be given for this towards the end of the course, as should time be given for both participants and trainers to say goodbye to each other properly. Trainers will need to assess what is appropriate, even if this means a time period for individual goodbyes to be said.

Course 1

Table 8.1 Timetable for a 2-day residential course on training the trainers for drug workers: part 1

	Day 1		Day 2
10.00 a.m.–11.00 a.m.	Session 1 Arrival, introductions 'What I'd like to learn'	9.30 a.m.–11.00 a.m.	Session 6 Plenary review of small-group exercise
11.00 a.m.–11.30 a.m.	COFFEE		
11.30 a.m.–1.00 p.m.	Session 2 'The structure and content of training'	11.30 a.m.–1.00 p.m.	Session 7 'The problems of planning and co-designing a course'
1.00 p.m.–2.00 p.m.	LUNCH		
2.00 p.m.–2.30 p.m.	Session 3 'What you need for a day's course'	2.00 p.m.–4.30 p.m. (with teabreak)	Session 8 Workshops
2.30 p.m.–5.30 p.m. (with teabreak)	Session 4 'Organising, designing and presenting a course' (small-group exercise)	4.30 p.m.–5.00 p.m.	Session 9 Course feedback – end of Part I
5.30 p.m.–7.30 p.m.	DINNER		
7.30 p.m.–9.00 p.m.	Session 5 'Organising, designing and presenting a course' (contd.) (small-group exercise)		

Finally it is worth reminding prospective trainers that learning is a two-way process, and that as trainers we can learn as much from participants as hopefully they can learn from us. We should never lose sight of this.

TRAINING THE TRAINERS – COURSE 1

Table 8.1 is one possible timetable for a 2-day residential course for up to eighteen drug workers with a 2-day follow-up, 3–4 months later.

The aim of this course is to help participants improve their existing training skills and to learn new ones.

COURSE FOR DRUG WORKERS

Part 1

Session 1

Following the Introductions, both to the course and to the other participants (Chapter 4, p. 65–6), the following exercise can be used as a method of focusing participants' thinking.

> **Exercise. 'What I'd like to learn'**   Participants are asked to write down individually on a piece of paper what they want to learn over the next two days (5 mins).
> They are then asked to *brainstorm* their answers which are written up on a flipchart by one of the trainers (10 mins). The flipcharts are put up on the wall and can be referred to throughout the course.

Session 2 'The structure and content of training'

This plenary session consists of three parts:

1 Presentation by the trainers on this topic using ideas based on, for example, Chapter 1 of this book or Cooper and Heenan's (1980) handbook (20 mins).
2 Discussion of these ideas and how these relate to participants' ideas and experiences (40 mins).
3 Participants can then either stay in the teaching room, or move

elsewhere to read individually a handout about 'co-designing' (see Appendix 8.5) (30 mins).

Session 3 'What you need for a day's course'

This short session should help people stay awake after lunch and start them thinking about the basic prerequisites of a course.

Exercise 'What you need for a day's course'   Participants are asked to *brainstorm everything* they will need to organise a course, from say, paper and pens to easily accessible toilets to external speakers. A trainer records this on flipcharts. This list can then be compared with the trainers' list shown on an overhead, and also given as a handout. (see Appendix 8.1 for a handout) (30 mins).

Sessions 4 and 5 'Organising, designing and presenting a course'

These two sessions based on a small-group exercise give participants the chance to organise, co-design and discuss how they would present a 1-day course for 24 people. It is useful to give a short presentation (10 mins) on workshop design at the start of Session 4. This can be based on, for example, pp. 107–12 of Cooper and Heenan (1980) and on your own experience. Then participants should be formed into small groups of three and each small group is given the details of a course to be designed (see Appendix 8.2 for examples. If the examples given in the Appendix are not relevant to the participants' situation, then you can design more appropriate ones.) If there are six small groups, then six different courses can be designed. Should there be more small groups, you may wish to duplicate courses in order to allow a chance for comparisons of design between two groups for the same course.

A resources table should be available to allow participants to consider different training materials. However, it should be stressed that the course design should be participants' own work which should be thoroughly discussed and, as far as possible, agreed upon by all members of each small group. Their course should be their own unique design.

Throughout these sessions one trainer should be available to answer questions. It is not necessary for trainers to facilitate the small groups.

Participants should be asked to write up their course design on flipcharts in preparation for Session 6.

Session 6 Plenary review

The completed flipcharts from Session 5 are displayed on the wall. Each group explains what attitudes, information and experience informs the design of their course and if there was consensus amongst the group members. Discussion. Participants should compare and contrast courses and should look at why one layout may suit one group but not necessarily another. This highlights the importance of designing the course around the group's needs.

Session 7 'The problems of planning and co-designing a course'

Participants are put in different small groups from the previous group and are given the chance to talk about the problems of co-designing and how these problems were resolved. As part of their discussion, participants should refer back to the handout on co-design with special emphasis on problems caused by stylistic differences, feelings, and responsibility.

It can be useful at this point for participants to go back into their original small groups from Sessions 4 and 5 so that they can talk about problems that arose with their co-designers.

A plenary session is also useful to air differences and to reassure people that co-designing, although the most effective way of offering training, has to be worked on to achieve results (30 mins).

Session 8 Workshops

These are based on two areas of drug training:

1 How to present an attitudes exercise to a small group.
2 How to make a presentation in front of a group of people.

This presentation can be videoed to enable participants to evaluate their own performance and constructively criticise others. Participants choose which workshop they want. Normally if there are two trainers, participants would only have time to try one workshop. However, if you have the time, the trainers and the video equipment, it would be possible to break into small groups and offer participants the opportunity to do a mixture of both workshops. Trainers should encourage participants to take a risk and involve themselves in a workshop which might at first glance appear threatening.

Workshop A   Participants are asked to choose an attitudes exercise (see Chapter 2) which they wish to practise using in a small group. Ideally each person should be given at least 15 minutes to present the exercise to the rest of the group, start them working on that exercise and, where possible, begin the discussion. Negative *and* positive feedback is then given by the trainer and workshop members as to how they felt about this presentation. The trainer should also act as timekeeper.

Here is some feedback which may be relevant during this workshop:

1 It is very important to test out exercises before using them with a small group. Sometimes trainers may use exercises they have not experienced themselves, or have not tested out on co-workers; this means they cannot anticipate any problems surrounding the use of the exercise.
2 Testing out exercises before using them allows you to make mistakes and therefore to work out how to rectify them before the course. It is also worth talking to other trainers about the benefits and problems of specific exercises.
3 It is important to be clear in the instructions you give to a group as to what they are expected to do, or how to complete the task or exercise.
4 Try creating a comfortable atmosphere for the group to work in. Think about the temperature of the room, the seating. Are people sitting in a circle? Can they see each other? Do they need a window open? Is the sun shining into someone's eyes? Has everyone been introduced to each other? Have you introduced yourself to the group?
5 Understand that groupwork skills can be applied in educational groups. This relieves the feeling of being deskilled which some participants may feel, who would otherwise be very comfortable in task or therapy groups. Therefore, be aware of the content and process of the educational group.
6 Do not be overenthusiastic to give the group the 'answers'. Small groups can be very skilled at inflating the ego by playing to the

'expert' in you. Be prepared to put questions back to the group to discover the knowledge they have within themselves. Also give the group time to find out what knowledge they have; do not rush in with the correct answer.

7 Encourage all group members to participate.

8 Be careful of the timing. As group tutor you are the person responsible for keeping the group to time to fit in with the rest of the course.

9 Be yourself. You do not have to adopt a role or new persona just because you have become a small group tutor. If you are relaxed and yourself then the group members will feel more comfortable and more able to express themselves.

Workshop B   Participants are asked to give a 5-minute presentation on a subject of their choice using visual aids, such as an overhead projector, if they wish. This presentation is videoed by the trainer, whilst the other workshop members act as the audience. The video is then played back. Feedback is given by the trainer and other workshop members as to how they felt about the presentation, both positive and negative. Trainers should be sensitive to any potential embarrassment that presenters may experience when seeing themselves on video. Remember to allow time for preparation of the talks before any presentations are videoed. This workshop needs to be strictly timed by the trainer. Here is some feedback which may be relevant during this workshop:

1 The introduction of any talk is very important. This is the first impression your audience will probably have of you. What impression do you want to create? Do you put them at their ease? Are you contentious? Do you make them laugh? Are you using language they cannot understand? Have they gone to sleep already? Be aware of how you come across to others.

2 Learn how to use correctly any audio-visual aids you may use during the presentation otherwise your talk will appear amateurish and badly prepared. For example, do not stand directly in front of the flipchart or overhead projector. Make any writing clear and legible and slides/overheads should be in focus.

3 Be aware of any nervous habits you may have which can be off-putting to an audience. What do you do with your hands? Do you frequently punctuate your talk with 'ahs' or 'uhms'? Do you sometimes put your hand over your mouth when talking due to

nerves? Note your positioning and posture. Do you move from one foot to another?

4 Does your voice carry to everyone in the room? Possibly your voice will become quieter or louder because you are feeling nervous. It is all right to ask if everyone can hear what you are saying, even if you are using a microphone.

5 It is important to prepare and rehearse the content of any talk you are to give. This may take time but is well worth it. It is unwise to write out the whole presentation verbatim. If you lose your place, this will cause you confusion, or you may be tempted to read it word for word, thus ensuring no dialogue or communication with your audience. Try instead using various types of *aide mémoire*, e.g. written cards, overheads, key words.

6 Watch the time. Have a watch handy, or make sure you can see a clock on the wall. If all else fails, ask someone to tell you when you have 5 minutes left, and then when your time is up.

7 Do not be too critical of yourself. It is easy to be very critical when you see yourself videoed for the first time, but use this as a means to an end. The more you practise, the more confident you become, and the more able you are to relax and be yourself.

Session 9 Course feedback

See Chapter 1, p. 11 on evaluation. You may also ask for specific feedback on what participants want included in Part 2 of the course.

Part 2

The aim of this follow-up is to review what was learned on the first part of the course and to offer participants time to practise their training skills.

Session 1 Welcome and review

A questionnaire (see Appendix 8.3) is distributed to participants which they complete individually (10 mins). Participants then go into small groups of three to discuss the answers to the question-naire (40 mins).

Table 8.2 Timetable for a 2-day follow-up course on training the trainers for drug workers: part 2

Time	Day 1	Time	Day 2
10.00 a.m.–11.00 a.m.	Session 1 Welcome and review	9.30 a.m.–11.00 a.m.	Session 5 Practical work (contd.)
11.00 a.m.–11.30 a.m.	COFFEE		COFFEE
11.30 a.m.–12.45 p.m.	Session 2 Review (contd.) planning practical work	11.30 a.m.–12.45 p.m.	Session 6 Review of practical work
1.00 p.m.–2.00 p.m.	LUNCH		LUNCH
2.00 p.m.–6.00 p.m. (with teabreak)	Session 3 Practical work	2.00 p.m.–3.30 p.m.	Session 7 Course design 'Learning how others do it'
		3.30 p.m.–4.00 p.m.	TEA
		4.00 p.m.–4.30 p.m.	Session 8 Feedback – end of course
6.00 p.m.–7.30 p.m.	DINNER		DINNER
7.30 p.m.–9.00 p.m.	Session 4 Practical work (contd.)		

Session 2 Review continued

This is a plenary session reviewing participants' answers to the questionnaire. It is important to look at what *helped* and *hindered* participants using what they learned on the first part of the course. The rest of this session is used to organise Sessions 3, 4 and 5.

Sessions 3, 4 and 5 Practical work

Ideally three trainers should be used here working with small groups of six. Each group should have a room large enough for presentations to be videoed. The practical work consists of:

1 Dealing with difficult group members.
2 Presenting 'Drugs and their effects' using visual aids. This is videoed.

Where possible all participants should have an opportunity to practise both 1 and 2.

Dealing with difficult group members

Beforehand, prepare cards with cameo descriptions of the behaviour of twelve difficult people you might find in groups, one description per card. If you cannot think of twelve problematic types of behaviour from your own experience, then either ask for ideas from participants during Session 2, or use some of the following examples. Here are a few ideas:

1 The 'know-it-all'.
2 The person who never speaks.
3 The person who constantly interrupts others.
4 The person who looks out of the window all the time.
5 The person who reads the handouts instead of participating.
6 The person with set views who is not interested in other people's opinions.

Using the attitudes exercise of their choice (see Chapter 2) each participant is given at least 15 minutes to present that exercise to the rest of the group, start them working and begin the discussion. The trainer hands one card each to two of the group who will play the parts of the difficult group members throughout this exercise. All the other participants are handed a card saying they should be themselves. Remember to debrief the 'difficult' members by asking them who they are, where they are and what they are doing before moving on to the next participant's attempt to deal with two difficult group members. This exercise is fun and everyone should have a chance to be a difficult group member. Apart from the briefing, debriefing and feedback, the trainer's role here is one of observer and timekeeper.

After the allotted time negative *and* positive feedback is given by the trainer and group members as to how the group was facilitated.

Here is some feedback which may be relevant during this workshop:

1 Remember the feedback mentioned following Workshop A (p. 161–2) in the first part of the course. This is all pertinent when dealing with difficult group members.
2 Group tutors may need to learn more about body language in order to anticipate potential problematic group members. Particularly when people are not talking in a group, their body language may say what the problem is.
3 Do not challenge or intervene every time the difficult group member speaks. It may be more appropriate for the other group members to respond and deal with the problematic attitude or behaviour. Anxiety can make you feel obliged to intervene in an attempt to sort the matter out. Encourage the other group members.
4 Try to understand what may be the underlying reason for the problem. Is it that the person simply does not want to be there? Have they been sent there by their manager against their wishes? Is there a football match, or other attraction on the television which they would rather be watching? Do they disagree with what is being said but are not assertive enough to say so? Did they have a quarrel with their lover last night?
5 It is important to try and reinforce any positive behaviour within the group rather than constantly referring to the negative behaviour. This in itself may encourage other group members to resolve the problem for themselves.

It is also useful to discuss with the group members how they would deal with the different behaviours mentioned on page 165. Here are some ideas adapted from Cooper and Heenan (1980):

The Know-it-all. This person wants to be seen as the resident expert. Whatever is said he or she will add to it or correct it, and is constantly seeking recognition and power. Such behaviour is an attempt to discredit the group leader, so avoid an argument at all costs. Suggest such persons offer their standpoint later to the group, and, as they have already had a chance to put their views, that they might like to allow others time and space now. You could suggest that they give a presentation to the whole course later on; this can be a suggestion put to the other course members. Ask why they have come on the course given they know so much. Suggest they discuss this with you at the end of the workshop.

The Withdrawer. This person may look out of the window all the time, or may choose to read his or her handouts, or at worst a newspaper, rather than involve him/herself in the group. He or she may look miserable and will be obviously distracted. The group members will usually be aware of this person and their feelings even if they are quiet and this can have an unsettling effect on them. This person needs to feel safe, and should be encouraged to express his/her feelings. He or she may be feeling very insecure or very negative about the experience. Should the behaviour continue then the group leader needs to challenge such persons individually and preferably away from the rest of the group. Ask them if they are dissatisfied and how they would like to change what is happening in the group.

The Monopoliser. This person constantly interrupts the other group members and is a poor listener who is not good at letting others express their point of view. Other group members may challenge him/her but the group leader should encourage the total group to deal with this by saying, for example, 'I am interested in other people's viewpoint; maybe those of you who have not had a chance to say anything yet would like to tell us what you think.'

Presenting 'Drugs and their effects'

Participants are asked to present the first 10 minutes of a talk on 'Drugs and their effects' using the overhead projector and, if necessary, the flipcharts. This is videoed. The aim of this exercise is not only to watch and listen to the presenter's style and material, but also to see whether they can effectively use visual aids. Before all the presentations are videoed, participants should be given enough time to write their talks and prepare their overheads. This means that the talks can be given one after another, and those who go first are not disadvantaged over those who make their presentations towards the end. If participants have not used an overhead projector before, then you may need to include some instruction on this in Session 2.

Whilst the trainer is videoing and timing each presentation, the other group members act as the audience. It is worthwhile videoing their reactions, as body language at the time may say more about how interesting the talk really is than comments made later. The video is then played back, and both negative *and* positive feedback is given by the trainer and the audience. It is important to take account of how the presenter feels about their performance.

Session 6 Review of practical work

To review the practical work you should carry out the following exercise:

> **Exercise 'How I felt about the practical work'**   In pairs, participants are asked to take time out, e.g. by going for a walk, to discuss how they felt doing the practical work, what problems arose for them and what insights they have had about their training skills (45 mins). Participants then return to the plenary for a general discussion about the above (30 mins).

Session 7 'Learning how others do it'

Participants go into small groups to discuss what training materials they are using in their current training work, how they are using them and how effective they think they are. Trainers can facilitate these groups, adding their own advice and learning to that of the course members.

Session 8

See Session 9, Part 1, p. 163.

TRAINING THE TRAINERS COURSE 2

Table 8.3 is one possible timetable for a 2-day residential course for up to twenty-four trainers who want to learn about drug training.

Note. If they have no knowledge of 'Drugs and their effects', then

Course 2

Table 8.3 Timetable for a 2-day residential course for trainers who want to learn about drug training

	Day 1		Day 2
10.00 a.m.–11.00 a.m.	Session 1 Arrival, introductions – 'The philosophy behind drug training'	9.30 a.m.–11.00 a.m.	Session 6 'Designing a 1-day basic drug course' Course content
11.00 a.m.–11.30 a.m.		COFFEE	
11.30 a.m.–1.00 p.m.	Session 2 'What are the problems?'	11.30 a.m.–1.00 p.m.	Session 7 Course content (contd.)
1.00 p.m.–2.00 p.m.		LUNCH	
2.00 p.m.–4.00 p.m. (with teabreak)	Session 3 'The importance of tackling people's attitudes'	2.00 p.m.–4.00 p.m. (with teabreak)	Session 8 Workshops
4.00 p.m.–5.30 p.m.	Session 4 'Local/regional analysis of drug use'	4.00–4.30 p.m.	Session 9 Course feedback – end of course
5.30 p.m.–7.00 p.m.		DINNER	
7.00 p.m.–9.00 p.m.	Session 5 'How to present "drugs and their effects"'		

a 1-day Drug Awareness Course should precede these 2 days.

Although there is no follow-up timetable, where appropriate you may wish to bring participants back together for a 1-day review.

The aim of this course is to help participants understand the philosophy behind drug training and how this can be applied when designing a drug course.

COURSE FOR TRAINERS

Session 1 Arrival, introductions – 'The philosophy behind drug training'

Following the introductions, both to the course and to the other participants a trainer should give a 15/20 minute input on the philosophy behind drug training. Ideas for this can be taken from various chapters in this book or other sources. Time should be allowed for a brief discussion.

Session 2 What are the problems doing drug training?

This session will give participants an opportunity to discuss their possible fears and worries about doing drug training.

1 Participants are asked to write down individually what their fears and worries are about doing drug training, and what they see are the problems (10 mins).
2 In small groups of six, participants are asked to share their individual thoughts, and to identify three major fears/worries/ problems common to group members to bring to the plenary session (50 mins).
3 Plenary session. Each small group talks about their three problems; these are discussed, then written on a flipchart by a trainer, pinned to a wall, and can be referred to throughout the course (30 mins).

Session 3 The importance of tackling people's attitudes

Before dividing into small groups, participants should be reminded why it is important to tackle people's attitudes to drugs and drug users. (This should have been fully covered in Session 1). If using three trainers, then each trainer can present a different attitudes exercise (see Chapter 2) and the three small groups can move round each trainer sampling the exercises. Thirty minutes should be given for each exercise so that groups move round at the same time. Participants can then go back into the plenary for a general discussion about the value of each exercise.

Session 4 Local/regional analysis of drug use

This exercise is a useful way of checking out what participants' knowledge is of their local drug problems. It also helps clarify what is substantiated factual information, and what is not. Participants are given a chance to verify that information with other participants and to ascertain what useful agencies can be used to collect information from in the future.

1 Participants are put in pairs or threes with others who work in the same area as them, i.e. who work in the same locality, district, or region. They are then asked to graphically depict on a flipchart what the incidence of drug use is in their area. This can be illustrated in any way they choose. On a separate flipchart they should list all the groups of people and agencies they know of who might expand their knowledge of the incidence of drug use in their area (1 hour).
2 Plenary session. The completed flipcharts are displayed on the walls of the plenary room for other participants to see and they are encouraged to ask questions of each other. A brief check should be made by the trainers that no-one has any unanswered questions before ending the session (30 mins).

Session 5 How to present 'Drugs and their effects'

Ideas about how to present this session on a course are given in Chapter 3. The importance of this session is that participants have time to consider the alternative ways, and also have an opportunity to experience one of the small-group exercises, e.g. 'The costs and benefits of drugs' or 'So you think you know about drugs'. What you are aiming for is an increased confidence amongst participants that they can tackle this session on a course.

Sessions 6 and 7 'Designing a 1-day basic drug course'

Course content

The difference between these sessions and Sessions 4, 5 and 6 on
Part 1 of the course for drug workers is that, instead of concentrat-
ing on course design, in this exercise participants should be simply
considering the course content. For this reason, the outline courses
are all different (see Appendix 8.4 for examples) in order that
participants will look more carefully at the needs of those coming
on each course and how that may affect the course content. Participants should work in threes and, where possible, the same
course should be given to two small groups in order that comparisons can be made. The course content should be written on a
flipchart and presented to the plenary session at the end of Session
7. One hour should be allowed for this plenary session.

Session 8 Workshops

Workshops on specific areas of concern or interest should be
offered. This information can be elicited from participants prior to
the course. For example:

1 Drug education and the community
2 'Critical incidents' video (see Chapter 5)
3 Where to begin with HIV and AIDS training

Session 9

See Session 9, Part 1 of the Drug Workers Course, p. 163.

The aforementioned ideas and course outlines are just the
beginnings of the process of training to be a trainer in the drug
field. Managers, sponsors and workers can sometimes assume that
by sending someone on a 4-day course you can turn them into a
skilled trainer. This is not the case. It needs to be acknowledged
that good training styles, techniques and skills take years to
develop and perfect, in the same way that it takes years to become
a skilled counsellor, therapist or teacher. We believe that what
applies in the AIDS field also applies in the drug field: 'It is our
experience that training trainers to begin to develop comfort and
skills in teaching in these sensitive areas cannot be achieved by
alternative short-cut methods (such as cascade training) or in a

shorter period of time' (Cranfield and Dixon, 1990).

However, necessity may well dictate that drug workers and other people will have to provide training without much practice or related skills. While learning to be a trainer ideally takes a long time, realistically people also need to be empowered, enabled and supported to 'just do it!'.

Good communication and listening skills, for example, although intuitive in some people, need to be identified, structured and practised, along with an understanding of groups, before a person can become an accomplished and effective trainer. People learning to be trainers need not only training but also consultancy and supervision during their training practice to help them monitor and evaluate the development of their skills. Trainers who work in isolation, designing, planning and facilitating training events on their own, will not receive objective feedback from their peers or use other more experienced trainers as consultants to help them improve their courses. Receiving feedback solely from participants on training courses is unbalanced and trainers should actively seek feedback from others about their course designs, administration and training style.

Co-designing and consultancy is to be encouraged for even the most experienced drug trainer, as are trainer support groups where members can share and exchange ideas, receive constructive criticism and create supportive networks.

We would like to encourage those who undertake drug training to take account of these points, and indeed the guidelines to good training practice in the drug field set out in this handbook. Most of all we hope that training to be a trainer is a positive and enjoyable experience that you can share with the participants on your training events.

APPENDIX 8.1 WHAT YOU NEED FOR A DAY'S COURSE

Venue

Right size rooms; good lighting; windows; right temperature (enquire about heating/ventilation); enough rooms close together for small groups; no external noise; disabled access to all facilities; crèche facilities if necessary; easily accessible toilets; tea/coffee and herbal teas available when requested; catering arrangements for both vegetarian and meat eaters; easy parking; map and clear directions; rooms clearly labelled and directions to them on notice board at front of building; registration person to welcome participants; seating arrangements – adequate, varied (not too hard, not too soft!); smoking room available if no-smoking venue (and vice versa); if residential, check comfort of bedrooms, whether single or shared, bathroom facilities, arrangements for security overnight.

Teaching aids

Audio system (if needed); overhead projector plus foils and pens; video plus film and TV; correct sockets; electricity supply, plugs and adaptors; flipcharts and pens; Bluetac; drawing pins; Sellotape; paper clips; drawing materials (if using art work); pencils and pens; scrap paper; rubber bands; name labels; participants' teaching packs including participants' list, timetable and handouts; all material for resources table; your own teaching notes and materials!; participants' list for registration purposes.
Ensure that you have costed the course to cover the following:

Venue cost
Catering cost
Tutors' fees and expenses
Administrative costs
Leaflets and handouts in teaching packs for participants
Your own expenses (if not included in above)

Send details of the course out well in advance and ensure that all participants have the final details and directions as to how to find the venue in good time.

APPENDIX 8.2 TRAINING THE TRAINERS COURSE

Exercise   Your project has been asked to organise and present a 1-day course on 'Understanding and working with drug users' for the following group of people:
An interdisciplinary group in your district consisting of:

three social workers
three intermediate-treatment workers
three community education workers
three police officers
three health visitors

two child psychologists
a doctor
a priest
a psychiatrist
two local councillors
a head teacher
a health board manager

At the end of the exercise you have to give the following information on three or more separate flipcharts:

1 Timetable/list of contents e.g.	Aims and objectives
	Exercises
	Handouts
	Reading list
2 Logistics e.g.	Venue
	Number of rooms/meals
	Teaching equipment

3 Evaluation and assessment of course

Exercise   Your project has been asked to organise and present a 1-day course on 'Understanding and working with drug users' for the following group of people:
A community action group (who want to set up a drug project) consisting of:

three community activists
nine volunteers from local community (including 2 ex-drug users)
five parents of drug users
two community police officers
a social worker
a community education worker
a headteacher (primary)
a local doctor
a local councillor

At the end of the exercise you have to give the following information on three or more separate flipcharts:

1 Timetable/list of contents e.g.	Aims and objectives
	Exercises
	Handouts

2 Logistics e.g.
Reading list
Venue
Number of rooms/meals
Teaching equipment

3 Evaluation and assessment of course

Exercise   Your project has been asked to organise and present a 1-day course on 'Understanding and working with drug users' for the following group of people:
A family support group consisting of:

a social worker (group-liaison person)
fifteen parents of drug users
eight volunteers from the local community

At the end of the exercise you have to give the following information on three or more separate flipcharts:

1 Timetable/list of contents e.g.
Aims and objectives
Exercises
Handouts
Reading list

2 Logistics e.g.
Venue
Number of rooms/meals
Teaching equipment

3 Evaluation and assessment of course

APPENDIX 8.3 QUESTIONNAIRE

1 What training have you done since the first part of this course?
Specify _____

2 Did the first part of this course help you with this training?
If so, how?
If not, why not?

3 Have you found that the course helped you in any other areas of your work?

APPENDIX 8.4

Exercise   You have been asked to organise and present a 2-day residential weekend course entitled 'Understanding and working with drug users' for twenty-four part-time youth leaders from your area.

At the end of the exercise you have to give the following information on three or more separate flipcharts:

1 Timetable/list of contents e.g.   Aims and objectives
                                         Exercises
                                         Handouts
                                         Reading list

2 Logistics e.g.   Venue
                                         Number of rooms/meals
                                         Teaching equipment

3 Evaluation and assessment of course

Exercise   You have been asked to organise and present an eight-session evening course for a local education/prevention group from local communities. Those taking part are all local residents from a rural area within a radius of 15 miles. They are primarily interested in how to educate about, and hence prevent, an increase in drug use. The course will be entitled 'Understanding and working with drug users'.

The education/prevention group consists of:

a Church minister
a Roman Catholic priest
two district nurses
three community activists – all ex-drug users
ten local residents – all parents
six part-time youth leaders
a community education worker

At the end of the exercise you have to give the following information on three or more separate flipcharts:

1 Timetable/list of contents e.g.   Aims and objectives
                                         Exercises
                                         Handouts
                                         Reading list

2 Logistics e.g.   Venue

Number of rooms/meals
Teaching equipment

3 Evaluation and assessment of course

Exercise   You have been asked to organise and present a 2-day course entitled 'Understanding and working with drug users' for an interdisciplinary group in your district.
The group consists of:

three social workers
three intermediate-treatment workers
three community education workers
three police officers
three health visitors
two child psychologists
a doctor
a priest
a psychiatrist
two local councillors
a headteacher
a health board manager

At the end of the exercise you have to give the following information on three or more separate flipcharts:

1 Timetable/list of contents e.g.   Aims and objectives
                                        Exercises
                                        Handouts
                                        Reading list
2 Logistics e.g.   Venue
                                        Number of rooms/meals
                                        Teaching equipment
3 Evaluation and assessment of course

APPENDIX 8.5 CO-DESIGNING AND CO-PRESENTING A COURSE

Co-designing is recommended as a more positive way of working than designing and presenting a course by yourself. Although it can be more time consuming and, at times, can create more work, it is fun and rewarding, offering a more supportive method of planning and teaching courses.

Table 8.4 Some benefits and costs of co-designing and co-presenting/leading benefits

Benefits	Costs
Co-worker to bounce ideas off; to help improve and expand sessions	Need to accept differences of opinion as assets, not faults
Co-worker to share the responsibility for the course	Need to compromise – you cannot have it all your own way
Co-worker to give you support through the good and bad bits – a look, a smile, even a gesture can help if you feel stuck or deskilled	Beware of any breakdown in communication or unexpressed feelings being obstructive
Co-worker to debrief with at the end – to offer a different perspective	You may end up designing a course with someone who does not offer you support, or whom you dislike
Ideally, a co-worker to share the workload – both the practical and the administration	You cannot take all the credit for a good course
Co-worker to laugh and cry with before, during and after the event	If co-worker is lazy or impractical you may have to do all the administrative tasks yourself

You should also be aware of the following areas:
The need to trust co-workers.
The difference in thinking styles – for example, global and concrete thinking, i.e. general and specific. These can work well together if both are accepted as valuable.
Differing energy levels – these will fluctuate and change. When planning a course always have breaks to re-energise.
Being prepared to explore and share your feelings and being aware of how comfortable you are co-designing.

Adapted from: Cooper and Heenan, 1980: 49–56.

REFERENCES

Cooper, S. and Heenan, C. (1980) *Preparing, Designing, Leading Workshops – A Humanistic Approach*, New York: Van Nostrand Rheinhold.

Cranfield, S. and Dixon, A. (1990) 'Training trainers to teach on drugs and Aids', paper presented at the First International Conference on Reduction of Drug-related Harm, University of Liverpool.

De Haes, W.F.M. (1986) 'Drug education? Yes, but how?', background paper, Health Education Research Symposium, Addictive Behaviours, University of Dundee.

De Haes, W.F.M. and Schuurman, I. (1975) 'Results of an evaluation study of three drug education methods', *International Journal of Health Education* 18(4) (Suppl.).

Index